Ebony Notes for Black Women

Uplifting Words, Affirmations, and Actionable Steps for Black Women on the Path to Healing, Love, Friendship, and Self-Care

LaDonna Welch

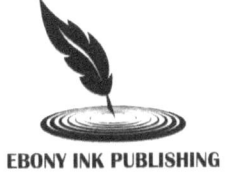

EBONY INK PUBLISHING

To request permissions, contact the publisher at
info@ebonynotesco.com

Hardcover: 979-8-9928756-0-7
Paperback: 979-8-9928756-1-4
Ebook: 979-8-9928756-2-1
Audiobook: 979-8-9928756-3-8

Library of Congress Number: 2025908403

First Edition: September 2025

Cover Art by LaDonna Welch
Headshot Photograph by Cat Salley

Ebony Ink Publishing

ebonynotes.co/pages/ebonyinkpublishing

This book is dedicated to the countless Black women who have made a positive impact on me. Your positive words, encouragement, advice when needed, and overwhelming support affected me in ways you'll never know.

To my girls, Skylar and Danielle, I hope I am doing a great job of showing, not just telling, you both that there is no limit.

Table of Contents

Foreword

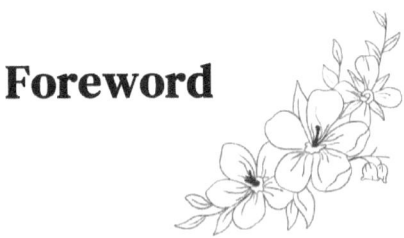

Dear Black Women,

I'm excited that you chose this book! It's an indication that you are intentionally choosing you, and that matters. I welcome you in all of your wonderful shades, personalities, fragrances, styles, creativity, and essences. You are fabulous! You're versatile and effortlessly dynamic. You are a force wrapped in what you determine is beauty. I recognize your greatness, but I also recognize that even the strongest of us need support. When was the last time someone asked about you and really waited for an answer? Having experienced a heartbreaking divorce and being a single mom of three young boys, there were times when I felt like the world was caving in on me. No one checked on me or my mental health to see if I were ok, not because they didn't care, but because they perceived that I had a "successful career" and I "held it together" so well. The truth was I could have used a "how are you today" and an opportunity to be real and vent. So today, I ask you...How are you today? No, really. How are you? Are you showing up right now as your authentic self, or are you doing good just to show up? Are you intentional about your thoughts, or are you paralyzed with overthinking? Are you displaying confidence in being you, or are you struggling with your self-image? Are you freeing yourself from over commitments, or are you carrying the weight of the world? Wherever you find yourself right now, know that you are not alone. If we are not currently there, we've all been there.

Circumstances and life, in general, can take us from one extreme to the next if we let them. I know the disappointments and demands life can bring, but I also know the joys and peace it offers. I "just existed" many days after my divorce, but books like this helped me gradually return to self, joy-filled and confident. And, I believe this book will do the same for you. It is full of ideas and advice to help you see you. It's here to help you learn to set boundaries and discover your importance, your deservedness, your entitlement to take care of self-first. When life is life-ing, this book will help you maintain.

Black Women, it's time to reclaim our joy, our peace, and, dare I say, our intentional focus on self, every day. We deserve it!

Yours in solidarity,

Dr. Danyell

No Penalties Just Promises®

Introduction
A Note from LaDonna

Hey girl hey! I'm LaDonna, and I'm thrilled to welcome you to *Ebony Notes for Black Women*—a journey into the heart and soul of Black women. This book is not just a collection of words; it's a sacred offering, a love letter to the women who move through this world with grace, strength, and confidence, even when the world tries to tell us otherwise.

I have been on a personal healing journey, and as I walk this path, I've come to realize that healing is not meant to be done alone. I want this book to be a companion for you, the way so many books have been for me. My mission is clear—to support the healing journey of as many Black people as I can, starting with us.

As I sit here writing these words, I'm filled with a mix of excitement, nervousness, and anticipation, nearing the completion of this book that has been a labor of love for over a year now. I am in my 16th year in the classroom—tired, a little burnt out, and ready to take a leap of faith into something new. It's a Sunday night, the clock ticking past 9:00 p.m., and there are only five more Mondays left in the school year. If you've ever counted down to the end of something, you know exactly how I feel! But even in the midst of my exhaustion, I still show up. I'm talking to God, seeking guidance, and trying to find balance—still waking up every morning to pour into my students, still mothering my own two babies, still striving to be the best wife, daughter, auntie, and sister I can be.

And yet, even with everything going on, I find myself drawn to this moment. This book. This opportunity to share something deeply personal with you.

Enough of that on that. So, why did I write this book? Why "notes" to Black women? And why is this mission so important to me?

Words Have Power

I have always believed in the power of words to uplift, inspire, and heal. Words shape the way we see ourselves and the world around us. I learned this at an early age, finding solace in books like *Chicken Soup for the Soul*—those little collections of stories that somehow made me feel less alone. Do you remember those books? I do, and I loved them. I had multiple! Did you?

They were comforting because they reminded me that someone, somewhere, had felt what I was feeling. That someone had been through the struggle and made it out on the other side. That's the kind of space I wanted to create with *Ebony Notes for Black Women*—a book filled with notes that meet you where you are, offering strength, encouragement, and a whole lot of love.

And this is just the beginning. I dream of *Ebony Notes* becoming a household name, with future books offering "notes" to Black men, teen girls, boys, grandmothers, fathers—our whole community. Because healing isn't just for us as individuals; it's for all of us.

Why Ebony Notes?

Let me tell you something funny—people call me Ebony all the time because of the name I chose for this company! And I get it. But *Ebony Notes* is so much bigger than me. The name carries meaning.

Ebony, a deep, rich shade of brown, represents us—the vast and beautiful spectrum of Blackness. It symbolizes our diversity, our history, our strength. It's a reminder that, despite our different backgrounds and experiences, we are connected. We share stories, struggles, and triumphs that deserve to be honored and heard.

Through *Ebony Notes*, I want to create a space where our voices are amplified, where our experiences are acknowledged, and where our stories are told with the depth and nuance they deserve.

Black Women Hold the World Together

As a Black woman, I know firsthand the weight we carry. We are often the foundation of our families, the glue that holds everything together. We take care of everyone—our children, our partners, our communities—sometimes leaving little space for ourselves. We are expected to be strong, to push through, and to show up even when we're exhausted. And yet, we rise.

But strength is not just about endurance—it's also about knowing when to rest, when to heal, and when to pour into ourselves. That's what this book is about.

What You Can Expect

Each chapter of *Ebony Notes for Black Women* is designed to pour into you. You'll find:

- Personal Notes – Heartfelt letters written just for you, like a friend sitting next to you, reminding you that you are seen, valued, and loved.
- Reflections – Deep dives into the themes that shape our lives, from self-worth and love to healing and joy.
- Affirmations – Words to speak over yourself, to counter the negativity the world throws our way.
- Actionable Steps – Practical tools and strategies to help you put the words into practice. Because healing isn't just about inspiration—it's about transformation.

You'll notice that some themes show up more than once, and that's intentional. Some things need to be said more than once because they are just *that* important. Repetition is how we unlearn harmful beliefs and replace them with truth.

My Hope for You

Sis, my hope is that this book meets you exactly where you are. That you find comfort in these pages. That you feel held. That you walk away from this book with a little more clarity, a little more confidence, and a whole lot of self-love.

You are not alone in this journey. There is a community of Black women—past, present, and future—who are walking this path alongside you. So, let these words remind you of who you are. Let them lift you when you feel low. Let them empower you to take up space, to rest without guilt, and to pursue joy relentlessly.

Welcome to Ebony Notes for Black Women

Here, your story is celebrated. Your voice is heard. Your journey is honored.

Let's begin.

With Love,

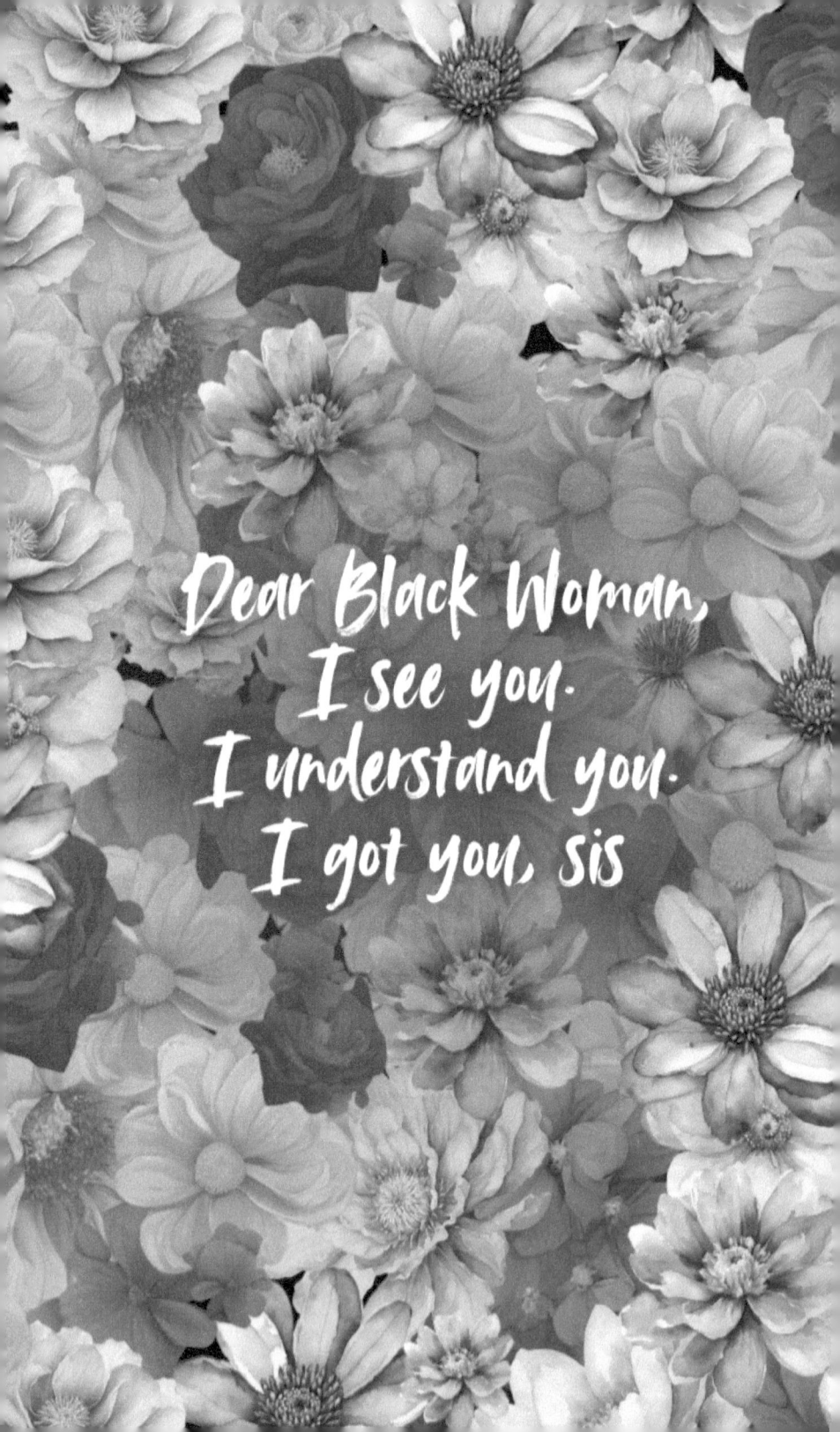

1

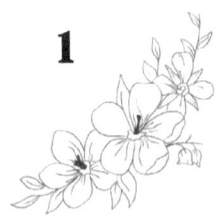

Starting with You: Finding Your Inner Goddess

Dear Beautiful Black Woman,

I'm here to tell you that you are a goddess. If you already know this, AYEEEE! I hope you are walking in your purpose. If you have not come to realize this yet, I'm here to make it plain for you. According to Merriam-Webster, a goddess is a woman whose great charm or beauty arouses adoration. In this modern day, a goddess is the representation of all that is divinely feminine. She is the embodiment of the powerful and nurturing energy of the Earth Mother, and is present in all living beings. The energy of the goddess, known as Gaia, is abundant and ever-flowing, like a beautiful river of grace. It is a blessing to connect with the goddess energy, for it is the source of all creation and healing.

You are a goddess, sis. You embody not only strength, tenacity, and wisdom but also beauty. You have overcome so much with grace that others can not show. You deserve to be celebrated and honored. Your courage and faith have brought you through every challenge, and you never give up. You have shown us that anything is possible and that our dreams can be achieved. Your presence in this world is a reminder of the power of love and fortitude. You are an inspiration to us all.

Starting with You: Finding Your Inner Goddess

You have the courage to stand up and speak your truth, the tenacity never to give up, and the compassion to share your love with those around you. You have the power to create, to heal, and to bring positive change to the world. Your beauty radiates from within and without, and your unique gifts are a blessing to us all. As a Black woman, you are a ray of hope and a source of inspiration. You are an amazing example of how strength and grace can co-exist. Your courage and strength are undeniable, and I honor you for all that you do. You are a goddess, and you deserve to be celebrated!

With love and admiration,

Your Inner Goddess

How is it that Black women carry the weight of careers, caregiving, and societal expectations—yet we continue to rise? It's undeniable that we carry a hefty burden, balancing demanding careers, extensive caregiving responsibilities, and the relentless pressure of societal expectations. Despite these challenges, we continue to defy the odds and rise above adversity. This resilience is a testament to our unwavering strength and determination.

Statistical evidence supports the notion that Black women are among the most educated demographics in the United States. This remarkable achievement underscores our commitment to intellectual growth and self-improvement. However, despite our educational attainment, we still face a persistent struggle for the respect and recognition that we rightfully deserve. This disparity highlights the deeply ingrained biases and systemic inequalities that continue to plague society.

In the face of these obstacles, Black women continue to thrive and flourish. Our ability to overcome adversity and achieve success is a testament to our inner strength and self-sufficiency. This remarkable capacity to persevere and excel, even in the face of daunting challenges, can be attributed to what can only be described as "goddess energy."

Looking within is the first step in shifting our thinking and belief system. It requires us to be honest with ourselves and acknowledge any limiting beliefs or negative thought patterns that hold us back. When we shine a light on these areas, we can challenge them and replace them with positive affirmations and beliefs.

As Black women, we come from a legacy of strength, independence, and innovation that has shaped history. We are worthy of love, success, and happiness—not because we have to prove ourselves, but because it is our birthright. Our power is undeniable, and our presence continues to inspire generations.

Our strength to keep going despite the odds has been an inspiration to many. Additionally, Black women are often praised for their unique beauty, intelligence, and ability to create vibrant, loving communities. All of these qualities combined make Black women deserving of the title "goddesses."

Too often, Black women are expected to be strong for everyone else, leaving little space to nurture our own needs and desires. But regaining your inner goddess means recognizing that you are more than the roles you fulfill for others—you are divine, powerful, and invaluable, just as you are. This shift in perspective is what Dr. Thema Bryant describes as healing the wounds of societal conditioning and stepping into our full power. She reminds us that our worth is not defined by productivity or sacrifice but by the undeniable truth that we are already enough. You are enough, sis!

Finding your inner goddess is all about tapping into your own power and strength. It's about connecting with the divine feminine energy that flows within each of us and using that energy to create a life that feels fulfilling and purposeful. To find your inner goddess, you must first look within and start shifting your thinking and belief system. As India.Arie sang in 'Video,' 'I'm not the average girl from your video / and I ain't built like a supermodel / But I've learned to love myself unconditionally, because I am a queen.' And you most certainly are a Queen. Her words remind us that beauty and worth are not defined by society's standards but by the love and acceptance we cultivate within ourselves.

Walk Through Fire, Emerge a Goddess

A goddess doesn't emerge from ease; she is shaped by fire. Sheila Johnson, co-founder of BET, is a testament to this truth. Her story is proof that goddess energy isn't just about radiance or confidence—it's about grit, reinvention, and the ability to forge something unbreakable from adversity.

You probably know BET, Black Entertainment Television, right? When people think of BET, they often think of Bob Johnson. But behind the success of Black Entertainment Television was Sheila Johnson—its co-founder and a driving force who helped shape the network into a powerhouse. Yet her journey wasn't without fire.

Sheila's life has been a masterclass in reclaiming one's power. Despite grappling with challenges such as struggles with conceiving children and facing her husband's abuse and infidelity, Shelia refused to let circumstances define her. Refusing to let societal limitations define her worth or dictate her destiny, she tapped into her inner goddess energy, rediscovered her power, and built her own legacy in a challenging professional landscape. Her path is truly inspiring.

Through sheer will and perseverance, Shelia shattered barriers and paved the way for future generations of Black women to follow in her footsteps. Her unwavering commitment to excellence and relentless pursuit of her dreams serve as an inspiration to all who dare to defy the odds and chase their passions. As the first Black female billionaire, Shelia Johnson stands as a beacon of hope and empowerment, a living testament to the transformative power of resilience, courage, and self-belief.

In her memoir, *Walk Through Fire*, Sheila reflects on the trials she endured—not just as a businesswoman but as a wife, a mother, and a Black woman in an industry that wasn't always welcoming. She shares:

"I had to learn that walking through fire is not about being consumed by the flames but about forging something stronger, something unbreakable within yourself."

Like Sheila, you, too, have the power to rise from difficulty, to walk through fire without being consumed by it. The flames will forge you, not break you.

Shelia's story is a powerful reminder that goddess energy is about more than beauty or confidence—it is about perseverance, self-reclamation, and owning your narrative. Sheila did not allow past hardships, including an abusive marriage and being overshadowed in business, to define her. Instead, she found the strength to reinvent herself, becoming the first Black female billionaire (yes, I'm repeating this because it deserves it's moment to shine) and a leader in industries beyond entertainment.

Her journey reminds us of our innate power to rise above adversity, with perseverance being the key to unlocking our potential.

She taught us that "no" doesn't mean never. "No" just means "not now."

Let us draw strength from Shelia's example and embrace the divine energy within us, trusting in our ability to overcome any obstacle and create the life we desire. In honoring the legacy of Shelia and other trailblazing women, we pave the way for our own success and empowerment, embodying the essence of the modern-day goddess.

When we talk about embracing our inner goddess, we're talking about summoning that same fire within us—the ability to rise from difficult circumstances, to say *no* when something no longer serves us, and to boldly step into our power. As Sheila's story reminds us, no setback is final, and no obstacle is insurmountable when we fully embrace our worth.

Take this Affirmation from Sheila Johnson's Journey:

"No doesn't mean never. No just means not now. I walk through the fire knowing I am being shaped into the woman I am meant to be."

Borrowed Beauty

There is a profound connection between the historical imitations of Black women and the timeless archetype of the goddess. Just as the goddess embodies strength, wisdom, and beauty, Black women have been revered for these very qualities throughout history. However, this admiration has often been overshadowed by attempts to appropriate and commodify our likeness.

Throughout history, Black women's bodies have been both revered and exploited, our unique features and styles often co-opted by mainstream culture. One such example is the adoption of bustles during the Victorian era, which borrowed from our bodies and reshaped to align with Eurocentric ideals of femininity, which historically ignored or rejected the natural shapes and attributes Black women possess. The tragic case of Saartjie Baartman, a Khoikhoi woman from South Africa, epitomizes this exploitation. In the early 1800s, Baartman was paraded across Europe, ogled for her curvaceous body, and subjected to degradation because of a condition called steatopygia, which causes the accumulation of fat on the buttocks and thighs—traits that are naturally prominent in some African women. Saartjie's suffering and objectification gave birth to a trend rooted in humiliation, and her exploitation helped fuel harmful beauty ideals that still plague us today.

This was more than just cultural appropriation—it was the commodification of our pain. The world has always sought our *rhythm*, but it has never truly understood or embraced our *blues*.

In addition to fashion, beauty standards have also played a significant role in the appropriation of Black women's likeness. The use of lip plumpers and skin tanners by non-Black individuals reflects a desire to emulate our natural features. Yet, these attempts often result in caricatured representations that fail to capture the true essence of our beauty. Our obduracy shines through, embodying the divine essence inherent in our identity despite efforts to diminish our worth.

When you begin to embrace your own beauty, intelligence, and creativity, you step into the legacy of Black women who came before you—women who have thrived despite systemic barriers. The Harlem Renaissance, for example, was more than an artistic movement; it was a reclamation of Black identity and excellence. Writers like Zora Neale Hurston and artists like Augusta Savage used their craft to assert their power and challenge restrictive narratives placed upon Black womanhood. Hurston, unapologetic in her confidence, once wrote, *"I am not tragically colored. There is no great sorrow dammed up in my soul nor lurking behind my eyes. I do not mind at all."* Her words remind us that Black women have never been passive recipients of society's limitations—we have always defined ourselves on our own terms.

By recouping our narrative and embracing the goddess within, we honor the legacy of our ancestors and pave the way for future generations. The exploration of imitation and appropriation serves as a poignant reminder of the ongoing struggle for recognition and empowerment faced by Black women. By acknowledging the historical context of these practices, we regain agency over our narratives and celebrate the richness of our heritage. Through awareness and solidarity, we can resist erasure and embrace the beauty and strength of our community.

a Note from LaDonna

Now listen. Affirmations are truly my thing. If you have heard of Ebony Notes before now, you get my drift, but I rock with affirmations and think that they are truly powerful.

We are usually harder on ourselves and are our own worst critics. Think about something you did and how you reacted to the praise from others. I still have to stop myself from immediately speaking about what could have been better or what did not go as planned. In reality, no one would have even known those things if I had not said a thing.

I'm a work in progress, and I, too, am still growing in my goddess-hood, okay!

Affirmations

Affirmations aren't just feel-good phrases. They're rewiring your brain. Every word you speak to yourself carries weight, shaping how you perceive the world and, most importantly, how you perceive yourself. Affirmations are not just empty mantras; they are a powerful form of self-care, self-reclamation, and self-empowerment.

When spoken consistently, affirmations have the ability to shift not only your mindset but your entire reality. Studies show that self-affirmation activates the brain's reward centers, reinforcing positive self-belief and reshaping neural pathways. Essentially, when you affirm your greatness, your brain starts believing it, and that belief manifests in your actions, choices, and confidence.

As Black women, we carry a unique set of challenges; ones that often make it harder to embrace self-love and self-acceptance fully. We are expected to be strong, to hold it all together, and to pour into everyone else before we pour into ourselves. Over time, this conditioning can make self-doubt feel more familiar than self-celebration. That's exactly why affirmations are so important. They serve as a counter to the world's attempts to shrink us. They remind us of who we are, what we deserve, and what we are fully capable of achieving.

How to Use Affirmations

Affirmations work best when they are intentional and personal. The key is to choose affirmations that resonate with you on a soul level; ones that feel real, not forced. Here are a few ways to incorporate affirmations into your daily routine:

- **Say them out loud** in the mirror each morning as a way to set the tone for your day. There's power in hearing yourself speak positivity over your life.
- **Write them down** in a journal to reinforce them on paper. Seeing your words in your own handwriting deepens their impact.

- **Repeat them during meditation** or while practicing deep breathing to create a sense of calm and alignment.
- **Set them as reminders on your phone** so that throughout the day, you're greeted with affirmations of love and encouragement.
- **Use them as replacements for negative thoughts.** The next time self-doubt creeps in, respond with an affirmation that reminds you of your worth.

Affirmations and Science

While affirmations may feel spiritual, their power is backed by science. Research published in the *Psychology of Well-Being* journal by Cohn et al. (2014) supports the notion that self-affirmation can decrease stress and increase psychological resilience. When you consistently affirm yourself, you are, quite literally, restructuring your brain to believe in your own value. You are strengthening neural pathways that reinforce self-confidence and self-worth, making it easier to embody the woman you are becoming.

With this understanding, let's begin that transformation now.

Affirmations for Your Inner Goddess

Each chapter of this book will include affirmations tailored to the specific topic at hand. This is a *take what you need, leave what you don't* situation. Feel free to write them down, post them on your mirror, or share them with someone else who may need them. Let's start here:

1. I am worthy of love, respect, and success.
2. My melanin is beautiful and radiates strength and resilience.
3. I am powerful beyond measure and capable of achieving my dreams.
4. I honor my ancestors and the legacy they left behind.
5. I am worthy of abundance and financial freedom.
6. I trust the universe to guide me towards my highest good.
7. I am deserving of pleasure and joy in all aspects of my life.
8. My body is my temple, and I treat it with love and care.
9. I am a source of light and inspiration for myself and others.
10. I choose to live my life on my terms and embrace my authentic self.

Affirmations for Your Inner Goddess

The way we speak to ourselves determines the way we move through the world. When we speak with kindness, encouragement, and confidence, we create an energy that attracts the very things we desire. However, when we allow negative self-talk to dominate, we limit ourselves before we even begin.

Negative self-talk is not just a bad habit—it is a cycle that reinforces feelings of inadequacy and fear. If you constantly tell yourself you're not good enough, your brain will find evidence to support that belief. But when you replace those limiting thoughts with affirmations, you start rewiring the way you see yourself.

The world may not always affirm us, but we can affirm ourselves. We can take up space unapologetically, knowing that our voices, our beauty, and our power are undeniable. We have the ability to rewrite our narratives and reclaim our worth, and it starts with how we speak to ourselves. There is power in our thoughts and words. Mmkay!?!

Your Mindset is Your Superpower

This journey isn't just about saying affirmations—it's about believing them. It's about taking a closer look at your life and identifying where you've been holding yourself back. It's about challenging limiting beliefs and reminding yourself daily that you are enough.

When we shift our mindset, we shift our reality. We open ourselves up to possibilities we once thought were out of reach. We begin to see that what is meant for us is already on its way. And sometimes, all it takes is the decision to believe in yourself a little more each day.

Let this be your reminder: You are capable. You are deserving. You are powerful. And you can speak your dreams into existence—starting now.

Taking Action

Use the steps below to shift your mindset and embrace your inner goddess. There will be action steps in each chapter, and you may recognize a theme. Some action steps will be repeated as they are very, very important, sis!

o **Start each day with positive affirmations:** Write down five affirmations that feel right to you. Which one resonates the most today? Say it out loud. Begin your day by reciting those affirmations and empowering you to embrace your inner goddess.

o **Practice gratitude:** Take a few moments each day to reflect on the things you're grateful for. Cultivating a sense of gratitude can help shift your focus towards positivity and abundance.

o **Embrace self-care Routines:** Incorporate self-care practices into your daily routine, such as meditation, journaling, or pampering yourself with a relaxing bath. These routines can help you connect with yourself on a deeper level and nurture your mind, body, and spirit.

o **Surround yourself with supportive people:** Build a strong support network of friends, family, and mentors who uplift and encourage you on your journey of self-discovery and empowerment.

o **Set boundaries:** Establish healthy boundaries in your relationships and learn to say no to things that don't serve you. Protecting your energy is essential for maintaining your sense of self-worth and inner peace.

o **Cultivate self-love:** Practice acts of self-love and self-compassion regularly, such as treating yourself with kindness, practicing forgiveness, and celebrating your accomplishments, no matter how small.

o **Connect with nature:** Spend time outdoors and connect with the natural world around you. Nature has a way of grounding us and reminding us of our interconnectedness with all living beings.

o **Pursue passions and hobbies:** Explore activities that bring you joy and fulfillment, whether it's painting, dancing, writing, or cooking. Engaging in creative pursuits can help you tap into your inner creativity and express yourself authentically.

o **Seek growth and learning:** Challenge yourself to step out of your comfort zone and pursue opportunities for personal and professional growth. Whether it's taking a class, learning a new skill, or embarking on a new adventure, continuous learning can help you evolve and expand your horizons.

o **Celebrate your progress:** Take time to acknowledge and celebrate your achievements, regardless of their slightness. Celebrating your progress along the way can boost your confidence and motivate you to keep moving forward on your journey of self-discovery and empowerment.

Your femininity is sacred, and when you honor it, you awaken a power that has always been within you. In Yoruba spirituality, Oshun is revered as the Orisha of love, fertility, and flowing waters, embodying beauty, self-love, and abundance. As Thompson (1993) explains in *Flash of the Spirit*, Oshun's energy is a sacred force that represents the divine feminine, guiding those who honor her toward emotional fulfillment, creativity, and joy.

She teaches us that softness and strength are not opposites but complementary forces—two sides of the same divine energy. It is through this balance that we move through life with both grace and unshakable strength.

Like Oshun, you have the ability to attract joy, honor your worth, and flow with confidence in your own skin. You do not have to shrink or prove yourself meritorious—your existence alone is enough. When you embrace your inner goddess, you are stepping into a lineage of powerful Black women who have created, nurtured, and led, often in the face of adversity. Their strength flows through you, reminding you that you are not alone in this journey.

Finding your inner goddess is not about becoming someone new; it is about returning to yourself. It is about rediscovering the beauty, wisdom, and magic that have always been part of you. It is about breaking free from the constraints of societal expectations and standing fully in your truth, unapologetically.

So, if you're ready to start living a life of empowerment, start now. Take action using the steps outlined in this chapter. Speak your affirmations boldly. Take back your divine energy. And most importantly, give yourself permission to shine.

The world has been waiting for you to shine your light. Now is your time.

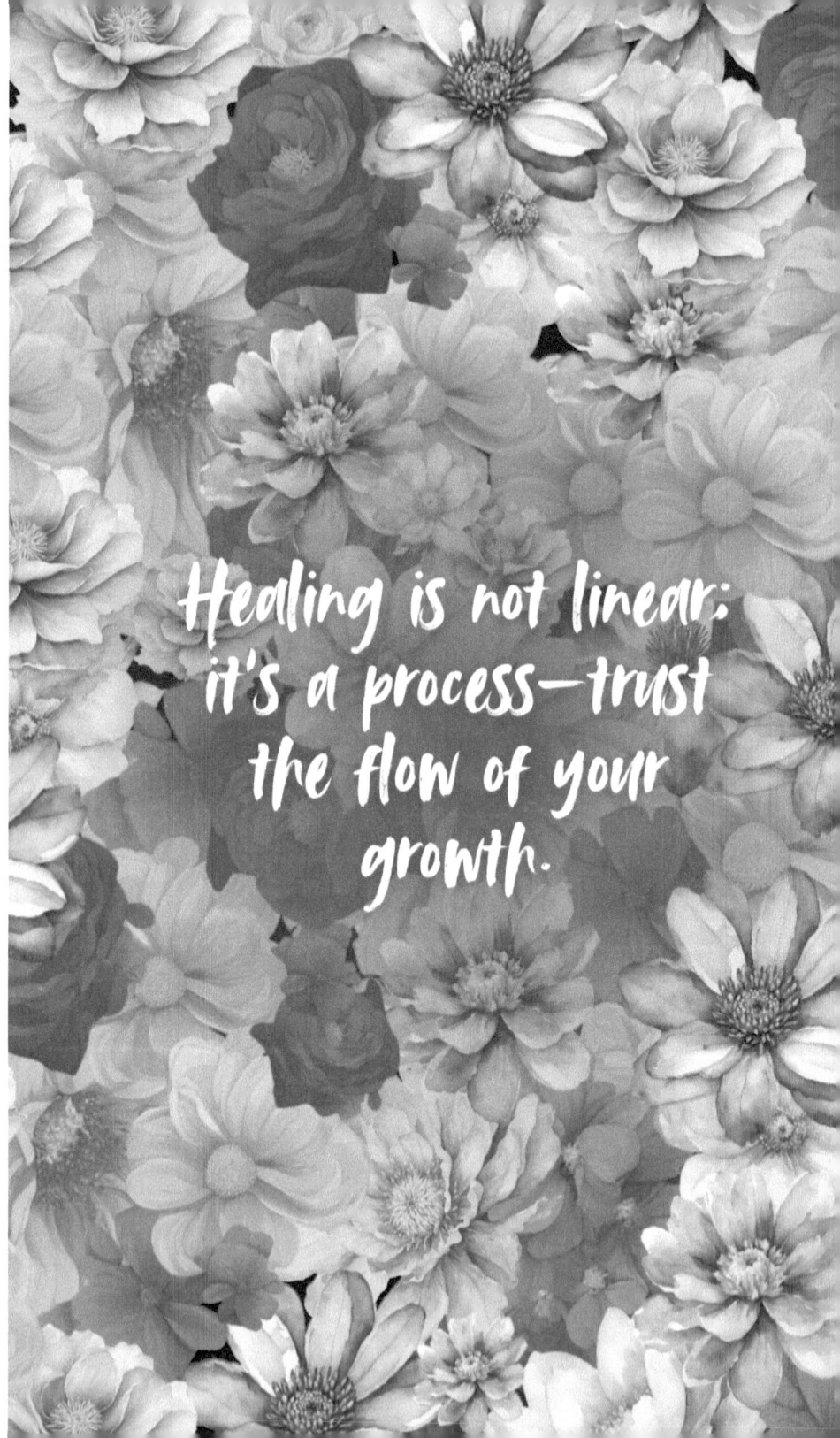

Healing is not linear;
it's a process—trust
the flow of your
growth.

2

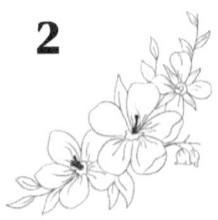

Healing for Black Women

To my Healing Sister in Arms,

I want you to hear something that is so important, so deeply ingrained in my heart, and I hope you'll listen with an open and loving spirit. You have permission to heal.

In a world that often demands so much from us, where the weight of expectations can bear down upon our shoulders, it's easy to forget that healing is not just a luxury——it's a necessity. It's not something that can wait for a more convenient time or when everyone else's needs are met. It's a fundamental right, and it's crucial to understand that healing is not selfish.

We, as Black women, are often the pillars of strength for our families, communities, and friends. We carry the weight of the world on our shoulders, and we do it with grace and persistence. But in the midst of caring for others, we must remember that we are not invincible. We are human, with our own needs, vulnerabilities, and moments of fragility.

Healing for Black Women

It's essential to recognize that healing isn't a sign of weakness——it's a sign of strength. It takes incredible courage to confront our pain, to tend to the wounds we've carried for far too long, and to seek help when we need it. The act of healing is an affirmation of your worthiness, a declaration that you are deserving of a life that is free from the weight of unresolved trauma and pain.

And here's a truth that I hold close to my heart: You cannot be the best version of yourself, the extraordinary pillar of strength if you are broken inside. You cannot pour from an empty cup, and your ability to help and uplift others is most potent when you, yourself, are whole and healed.

So, I implore you, don't deny yourself the opportunity to heal. Your healing isn't just for you, it's a gift to those you love, to your community, and to the world. It's the ultimate act of self-love and self-preservation, and it's an investment in your future well-being.

Remember, seeking help is a sign of wisdom, self-compassion, and strength. It doesn't diminish your role as a source of support and inspiration. On the contrary, it enhances it. It allows you to shine even brighter as a beacon of hope, a source of love, and an unwavering symbol of resilience.

So, take the time you need. Seek therapy, talk to trusted friends or family, or engage in self-care practices that nurture your spirit. You are entitled to the love and care you give to others, and it's time to extend that same love and care to yourself.

Stay Lifted,

Let's Begin the Journey to Healing

Healing is not simply a feel-good indulgence or a fleeting luxury reserved for those with ample time and resources. It is, in fact, a fundamental human necessity, as vital to our well-being as food, water, and shelter. Toni Morrison once wrote, *"If you surrender to the air, you can ride it"* (Morrison, 1977). Healing requires surrender—letting go of the need to have all the answers and trusting that you have a right to peace. Peace, Queen! It means giving yourself permission to unlearn the survival patterns that no longer serve you. It means believing that rest, joy, and wholeness are not rewards to be earned but birthrights to be claimed.

Black women have historically been the backbone of their communities, yet often, our healing is placed on the back burner. As Dr. Thema Bryant reminds us, *"Healing is not just about moving on; it's about reclaiming joy"* (Bryant, 2022). Many of us have been taught to equate strength with endurance, pushing through hardships while ignoring our own emotional and physical needs. But true strength lies in knowing when to rest, when to seek support, and when to allow ourselves the grace to heal. We are treasured and ready to heal in our soft girl era.

Healing encompasses a broad spectrum of experiences, from physical recovery and emotional restoration to spiritual growth and mental clarity. It is an ongoing process that requires attention, dedication, and self-compassion. Dr. Joy DeGruy, in her work on *Post Traumatic Slave Syndrome*, explains how the traumas of the past continue to affect Black people today. She highlights that healing is a collective effort, requiring not only personal introspection but also communal support (DeGruy, 2005). This means that when we embark on our healing journeys, we are also healing the generations before us and making space for those who come after us.

Whether we are recovering from a physical ailment, mending a broken heart, or grappling with the challenges of daily life, healing is essential for our overall health and happiness. Resmaa Menakem, author of *My Grandmother's Hands*, emphasizes that trauma is stored in the body, not just in the mind, and that healing must also be physical (Menakem, 2017). If you've ever felt tension in your shoulders from stress or exhaustion that won't fade no matter how much you sleep, your body is telling you that it remembers. Healing must happen not only in our thoughts but in how we treat ourselves holistically—through movement, breath, and intentional rest.

The journey towards healing can be a challenging one, but it is also one of the most rewarding and transformative experiences we can have. It involves taking a closer look at our past traumas and pain, acknowledging them, and seeking the support we need to move forward. bell hooks, in *All About Love*, reminds us that *"rarely, if ever, are any of us healed in isolation"* (hooks, 2000). Healing requires community, connection, and safe spaces where we can be heard and affirmed.

Therapy is one of the most effective ways to start the healing process. A skilled therapist can help us unpack our emotional baggage, identify our triggers, and develop coping mechanisms to deal with our past trauma. Therapy also offers a safe and non-judgmental space for us to process our emotions and work through our pain. Dr. Joy Harden Bradford, founder of *Therapy for Black Girls*, has built an entire platform dedicated to ensuring Black women can access culturally competent mental health professionals who truly understand their lived experiences (Bradford, 2017). Seeking therapy is not a sign of weakness; it is an act of self-preservation.

Another important aspect of the healing journey is finding a support system. Surrounding ourselves with people who love and support us can help us feel less alone in our struggles and provide us with a sense of belonging. Whether it's a close friend, family member, or a support group, having a support system can make all the difference in our healing journey.

Audre Lorde once said, *"Caring for myself is not self-indulgence; it is self-preservation, and that is an act of political warfare."* (Lorde, 1988). By prioritizing healing, we reacquire our power and assert that we have the right to care and restoration.

Journaling is another powerful tool for healing. Writing down our thoughts and feelings can help us gain clarity and insight into our emotions and experiences. It also provides a safe and private space for us to process our emotions and work through our pain. Dr. Gabor Maté, a trauma expert, explains that writing and self-reflection allow us to make sense of our past wounds and create new narratives that empower us rather than define us by our suffering (Maté, 2010). The simple act of putting pen to paper can be a transformative way to release pain and recognize growth. So write, sis. It'll help you heal.

Healing is not a luxury—it is a necessity. It is the foundation upon which we build the lives we truly deserve. By embracing this journey with intention, we affirm our worth, honor our ancestors, and create a legacy of well-being for those who come after us.

Journal Prompts

Get started with the prompts below, but if you ever need more, Pinterest, the Ebony Notes app, and https://ebonynotes.co/

have you covered (because, let's be real, we love options—shameless plug included!).

- Reflect on a time when you felt emotionally wounded or hurt. How did you cope with those feelings, and what steps did you take to heal?

- Think about the relationships in your life that may need healing. What actions can you take to address any lingering conflicts or tensions?

- Consider any past traumas or experiences that still affect you today. How can you begin the process of healing and letting go of these painful memories?

- Explore the role of forgiveness in your healing journey. Are there any individuals you need to forgive in order to move forward with your life? How can you practice forgiveness, both for others and for yourself?

- Think about the support systems you have in place for times of need. How can you strengthen these relationships and lean on them for support during difficult times?

- Consider any negative beliefs or self-talk patterns that may be hindering your healing process. How can you challenge these beliefs and replace them with more positive and empowering thoughts?

- Reflect on the progress you've made in your healing journey so far. What lessons have you learned, and what areas still require attention and growth?

♂ a Note from LaDonna

Let's chat about journaling, shall we? It's like having a secret weapon in your back pocket — your very own therapy session, no appointment necessary!

Now, I know what you're thinking: "But LaDonna, I don't have time for that!" Oh, girl, let me tell you, we make time for things that are important, and your healing journey is important.

Grab your pen (or keyboard, if you're feeling tech-savvy), and let's dive in. Pour out your thoughts, scribble down your dreams, and maybe even doodle a bit. Who says healing can't be fun?

And remember, on those tough days, just flip back through your journal and see how far you've come. You're stronger than you know, sis!

Breaking Barriers

Taraji P. Henson is a force both on and off the screen, using her platform to shed light on the importance of mental health in the Black community. Her transparency about her personal experiences with anxiety and depression has sparked critical conversations, challenging the stigma surrounding therapy and emotional well-being. In a society where Black women are often expected to be the strong ones, carrying the weight of the world with grace, Henson's openness serves as a powerful reminder that strength also means knowing when to ask for help.

In 2018, she took her advocacy a step further by founding **The Boris Lawrence Henson Foundation**—named in honor of her late father, a Vietnam War veteran who struggled with mental health issues. The foundation is dedicated to providing culturally competent therapy resources to Black individuals, addressing the barriers of access, cost, and stigma that often prevent us from seeking care. Henson's work highlights the necessity of normalizing mental wellness in our community and ensuring that resources are accessible to those who need them most.

By speaking candidly about her own journey, Taraji empowers Black women to give themselves permission to prioritize healing. She reminds us that seeking therapy is not a sign of weakness—it's a revolutionary act of self-love and self-determination. Her advocacy not only inspires but it also paves the way for more Black women to embrace therapy as a tool for growth, self-care, and generational healing.

Forgiveness

Let's chat about forgiveness.

Listen up, beautiful: forgiveness doesn't mean forgetting, and it certainly doesn't mean excusing someone's behavior. It's not about letting them off the hook—it's about freeing yourself. When you hold on to resentment, anger, or pain, it's like carrying around a heavy bag filled with bricks. Each hurt, each betrayal, each disappointment is another brick weighing you down. And sis, you were never meant to carry all of that.

So, let's take a deep breath together—inhale grace, exhale the weight of what no longer serves you. Forgiveness is about recovering your energy, your peace, and your power. It's about making the choice to stop allowing past wounds to dictate your present joy. Dr. Thema Bryant, a clinical psychologist and advocate for Black women's mental health, reminds us that forgiveness is a process, not a one-time event. In her book *Homecoming: Overcome Fear and Trauma to Reclaim Your Whole, Authentic Self*, she encourages us to see forgiveness as a step toward personal freedom rather than a favor to those who wronged us (Bryant, 2022).

Let's be clear: **forgiveness is for you.** It's not about saying what happened was okay. It's about refusing to let someone else's actions hold you hostage. You deserve to move forward without the burden of past pain clouding your path. So, give yourself permission to let go, to heal, and to make room for love, kindness, and peace. You've got this, and you are so worthy of the freedom that forgiveness brings.

In Our DNA

Our brother Kendrick Lamar was absolutely correct when he said, "I got loyalty, got royalty inside my DNA" (Lamar, 2017). Although he was correct, there is a lot more in our DNA. Generational trauma has had a profound and reverberating effect on our lives today. Our DNA carries not only the physical traits inherited from our ancestors but also the emotional scars of their experiences. Across generations, trauma can manifest in various forms, shaping our perceptions, behaviors, and responses to stressors.

Your body remembers what your mind tries to forget. As Dr. Bessel van der Kolk explains in The Body Keeps the Score, unprocessed trauma doesn't just live in our memories; it lives in our muscles, our nervous system, and our breath. That tension in your shoulders? The fatigue you can't shake? The anxiety that creeps in when you slow down? These are not just random aches; they are echoes of past wounds, asking to be acknowledged. This is why healing is not just emotional—it's physical. Movement, breathwork, and mindfulness can all help you release what your body has held onto for too long.

The history of slavery, segregation, and systemic oppression continues to cast a long shadow over our communities, leaving deep wounds that are often overlooked or dismissed. The trauma inflicted upon our ancestors echoes through time, leaving an indelible mark on our collective psyche. It informs our sense of identity, influences our relationships, and colors our view of the world.

In confronting the trauma of our past, we are confronted with the harsh realities of our present. The pervasive presence of racism, discrimination, and violence perpetuates cycles of trauma within our communities. The relentless onslaught of images depicting police brutality and racial injustice serves as a constant reminder of the systemic forces arrayed against us.

Yet, in acknowledging the pain of our past and present, we open the door to healing and transformation. Healing is not simply about overcoming adversity; it is about reclaiming our power, rewriting our narratives, and forging a path forward rooted in resoluteness and self-determination. By honoring our experiences, acknowledging our pain, and seeking support from our communities, we can begin the journey toward healing and wholeness.

You deserve to feel whole, to live without the weight of past pain. In All About Love, bell hooks remind us that 'rarely, if ever, are any of us healed in isolation.' Healing is not just an individual journey, it is communal. We need spaces where we can be heard, affirmed, and supported. Whether that means therapy, sisterhood circles, or simply granting yourself grace, the path to healing is one you don't have to walk alone.

Together, we can break the chains of intergenerational trauma, cultivate healing spaces, and build a future where our resilience shines brighter than our scars. Through collective action, self-care, and a commitment to justice, we can create a world where all Black women are empowered to thrive despite the challenges we face.

Taking Action

o **Be Kind to Yourself:**
  - o Set aside time each day to show yourself kindness and compassion.
  - o Practice positive self-talk and challenge negative thoughts or beliefs about yourself.
  - o Treat yourself with the same level of kindness and understanding that you would offer to a close friend or loved one.

o **Seek Support:**
  - o Reach out to trusted friends, family members, or professionals for support and guidance.

- ○ Consider joining a support group or seeking therapy to explore your emotions and experiences in a safe and non-judgmental space.
- ○ Surround yourself with individuals who uplift and encourage you on your healing journey.

○ **Prioritize Self-Care:**

- ○ Make time for activities that bring you joy and relaxation, such as spending time in nature, practicing yoga or meditation, or indulging in your favorite hobbies.
- ○ Take care of your physical health by eating nutritious foods, getting regular exercise, and prioritizing adequate sleep.
- ○ Set boundaries to protect your energy and well-being, and don't be afraid to say no to activities or commitments that drain you emotionally or physically.

○ **Practice Forgiveness:**

- ○ Work on forgiving yourself for past mistakes or perceived shortcomings.
- ○ Practice forgiveness towards others who may have hurt or wronged you, recognizing that holding onto anger or resentment only prolongs your own suffering.

- o Remember that forgiveness is a process and may take time, but it is essential for your own healing and growth.

- o **Embrace Healing Modalities:**
  - o Explore different healing modalities such as therapy, meditation, energy work, or alternative therapies like acupuncture or aromatherapy.
  - o Find what works best for you and incorporate it into your regular self-care routine.
  - o Be open to trying new techniques or approaches to healing, and trust your intuition to guide you toward what resonates with you.

- o **Cultivate Mindfulness:**
  - o Practice mindfulness techniques to stay present and grounded in the moment.
  - o Engage in activities such as deep breathing exercises, body scans, or mindful movement practices like yoga or tai chi.
  - o Use mindfulness to observe and acknowledge your thoughts and feelings without judgment, allowing them to pass without getting caught up in them.

- o **Connect with Your Inner Child:**

- Take time to connect with your inner child and nurture her needs and desires.
- Engage in activities that bring you joy and evoke a sense of playfulness and spontaneity.
- Offer your inner child love, comfort, and reassurance, allowing her to feel safe and supported as you navigate your healing journey.

- **Set Boundaries:**
  - Identify areas of your life where you may need to establish or reinforce boundaries to protect your emotional and mental well-being.
  - Communicate your boundaries clearly and assertively with others, and don't be afraid to enforce them if they are violated.
  - Remember that setting boundaries is an act of self-care and self-respect, and it is essential for maintaining healthy relationships and personal balance.

- **Practice Gratitude:**
  - Cultivate a daily gratitude practice by reflecting on the things you are thankful for in your life.
  - Keep a gratitude journal and write down three things you are grateful for each day.

o Focus on the positive aspects of your life and express gratitude for the lessons you have learned and the growth you have experienced.

o **Honor Your Journey:**

  o Remember that healing is a journey, not a destination, and it is okay to take things one step at a time.

  o Be patient and gentle with yourself, and celebrate your progress irrespective of dimension.

  o Trust in your ability to heal and know that you have everything you need within you to overcome any challenges that come your way.

Here are ten affirmations to help you on your journey toward healing:

1. I am deserving of healing and wholeness.
2. I release all negative emotions and thoughts that no longer serve me.
3. I forgive myself and others for past hurts and mistakes.
4. I am open to receiving the love and support I need to heal.
5. I trust in my own ability to heal and grow.
6. I am worthy of joy, peace, and happiness.
7. I release all shame and guilt associated with my past experiences.

8. I am resilient and capable of overcoming any obstacle.
9. I honor my feelings and give myself permission to feel and process them.
10. I am grateful for the healing journey and the lessons it has taught me.

Healing isn't easy, but it is necessary. You cannot move forward if you refuse to acknowledge the wounds that need tending. Dr. Joy DeGruy's research on Post-Traumatic Slave Syndrome reminds us that many of our struggles are not just individual—they are historical. The emotional burdens we carry are often passed down through generations, shaped by systemic injustice and cultural survival strategies. But recognizing this doesn't mean we must stay bound by it. Healing is our right. It is how we take back our wholeness, both for ourselves and for the generations that follow.

Ultimately, the journey toward healing is a deeply personal and individual one. It requires us to take an honest look at ourselves, acknowledge our pain, and seek the support we need to move forward. But with the right tools, support, and mindset, we can heal our wounds and start living a life of joy, peace, and purpose.

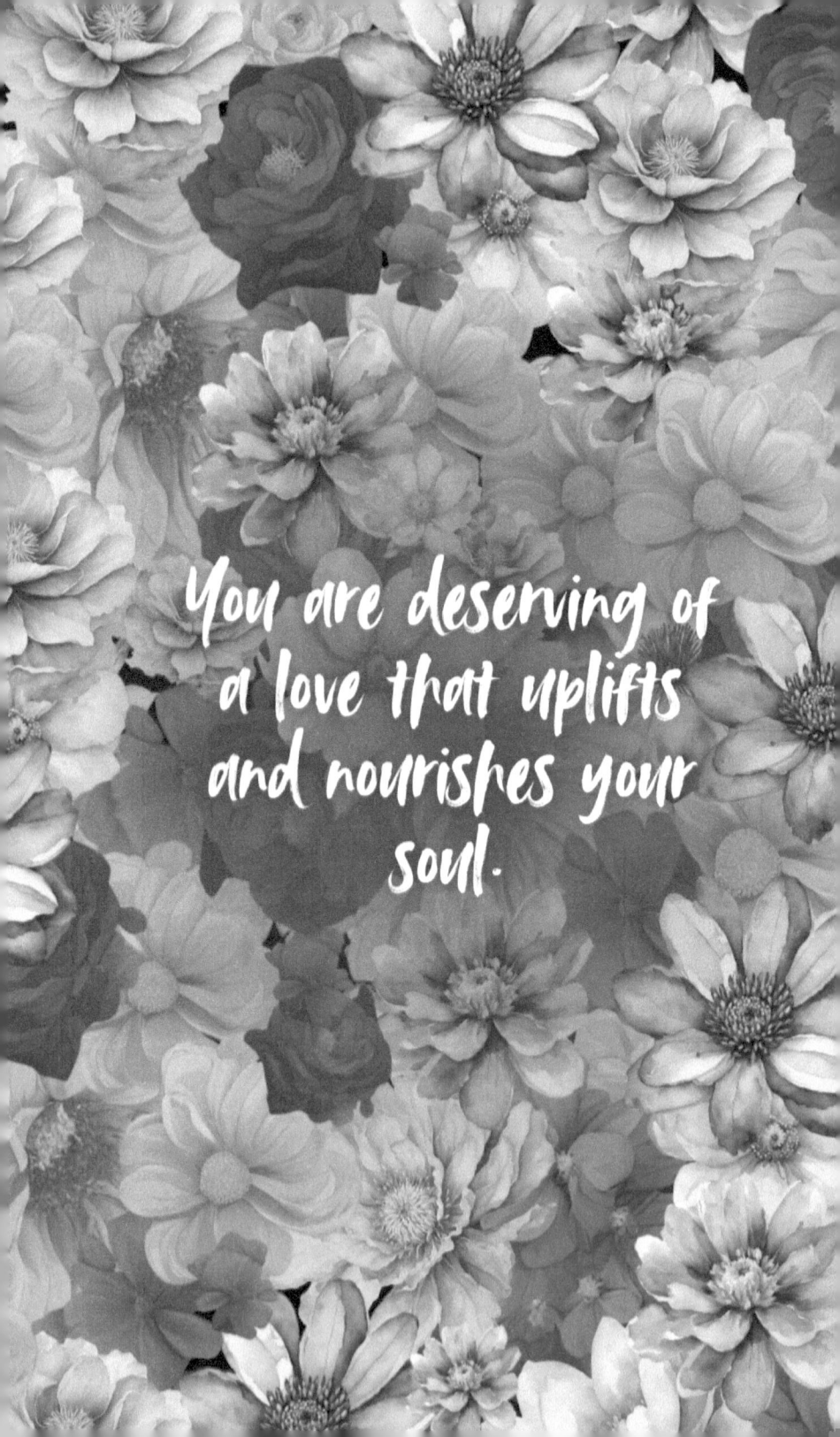

3

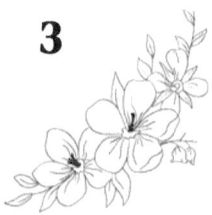

Love for Black Women

Hey there,

I want to remind you of something that lies at the core of our existence——love. Love is the universal force that binds us all together, and it comes in many forms. It is a force that we should extend not only to others but also to ourselves.

The song "Love" by Musiq Souldchild has always felt special to me. As a junior or senior in high school, I would sing this song at the top of my lungs, and baby not only did I not have a singing bone in my body, I had no idea what I was singing about at the time.

I remember a teacher discussing the song's meaning with me and a friend. As an adult, I revisited this conversation. Originally meant as a tribute to God, the lyrics express a deep desire to connect with love despite uncertainties. The chorus acknowledges love's complexities, as some misuse its name while others struggle with belief. Overall, "Love" captures love's power, struggles, and significance in shaping human experiences.

Love for Black Women

It's essential to recognize that love extends beyond oneself. It encompasses kindness, empathy, and understanding towards others. Love recognizes the humanity in every person encountered and chooses love even in the face of differences. It serves as the common thread that unites us all, transcending boundaries and fostering unity.

And remember, you deserve to be loved just as much as you love others. Don't settle for anything less than genuine, pure, and honest love. It's a gift that you give to the world, but it's also a gift you deserve to receive. Open your heart to the possibility of being loved fully, without reservation or compromise.

As you journey through the path of self-love and extend your heart to others, never forget that you are deserving of love in all its beautiful forms. Embrace the power of love, for it has the incredible ability to heal, transform, and create a world filled with compassion and understanding.

Keep on Lovin',

Introduction to Love

Love is the essence of who we are. It is a force that shapes our lives, influences our relationships, and impacts the world around us. As Black women, love is not just an abstract concept but a powerful, transformative energy that has carried us through centuries of struggle, potency, and triumph. In a society that often places heavy burdens on us, love is our lifeline, our reminder of our worth, and the foundation upon which we can build our peace.

But the journey to understanding and embracing love, true love, is one that starts within. It requires a deep connection to ourselves, a commitment to self-care, and a dedication to setting boundaries that protect our emotional, mental, and physical well-being. True love is not just about receiving affection from others; it's about nurturing the love we have for ourselves. This love serves as the compass that guides us in choosing relationships that uplift us, heal us, and inspire us to be the best version of ourselves.

Let's explore the many facets of love: romantic, familial, platonic, and most importantly, self-love. We'll delve into the complexities and beauty of love, reflecting on how we can cultivate it in our lives and how we can break free from past narratives that have limited our ability to receive and give love fully. Love is an ongoing journey, one that requires continuous nurturing, learning, and unlearning. A WORD! I'll just say that again. **Unlearning.**

I hope that you'll be empowered to embrace love in all its forms, heal from past heartaches, and open your heart to the boundless possibilities that love, both for yourself and others, can bring into your life.

True Love

Love is a powerful force that can bring us joy, fulfillment, and happiness. As Black women, we are often taught to put the needs of others before our own, and our experiences with love can be complicated and complex. We deserve to experience love in all its forms, but we also need to be mindful of the relationships we engage in and the impact they have on our lives.

Black women deserve the love that is safe, nurturing, and reciprocal. Too often, we have been expected to pour endlessly into others while receiving little in return. In *All About Love*, bell hooks reminds us that love is not just a feeling; it is an action. Love should not drain us; it should sustain us. It should be the foundation upon which we build our peace, not the reason we lose it. True love begins with the self, setting the standard for how we allow others to treat us. We should know that it is our responsibility to teach others how to treat us. As we learn to practice self-love, we pave the way for love to flourish in all other areas of our lives.

Love comes in many forms: romantic love, friendship, familial love, and self-love. It's important to acknowledge and appreciate all the love in our lives, whether it's from family, friends, or romantic partners. Each type of love can bring us joy and fulfillment, but it's important to recognize that not all relationships are healthy or positive. However, not all relationships are healthy, and it's crucial that we recognize and understand what healthy love looks like. As our girl Mary J. Blige sings, "Real love, I'm searching for a real love." Healthy love is built on respect, trust, communication, and mutual support, and it should lift us up, not drain us. It's important to acknowledge toxic relationships and the negative impact they can have on our emotional and mental well-being. We deserve the love that nurtures us, not love that diminishes our spirit.

Finding true love can be a journey filled with ups and downs, but it's important to stay true to ourselves and our values. It's important to take the time to get to know someone and establish a strong foundation of trust and respect before committing to a relationship. We also need to listen to our intuition and pay attention to red flags that may indicate a toxic relationship. This is where you use your power of discernment. Healthy relationships are not about fixing someone else's brokenness or tolerating unhealthy behaviors. It's about mutual growth, support, and respect. The Gottman Institute, known for its groundbreaking research on relationships, has found that emotional intimacy, effective communication, and empathy are key factors that predict long-lasting, fulfilling relationships (Gottman, 2017). Their work emphasizes that building and maintaining a healthy relationship is a continuous effort, requiring both partners to be willing to work through challenges with mutual respect.

Before we can truly love others, we must first love ourselves. We'll dive deeper into self-love later, but understand that when we love and accept ourselves, we attract partners who reflect those same values. It's important to set healthy boundaries and communicate our needs and expectations in relationships. By valuing ourselves and setting boundaries, we show the world how we expect to be treated.

Acknowledging and walking away from toxic relationships can be one of the hardest things to do, especially if we love someone deeply. But sometimes, walking away is necessary for our own growth and well-being. It's important to remember that we can still love someone from a distance and that walking away doesn't mean we don't care for them. It simply means that we care for ourselves enough to prioritize our own well-being and happiness. At the end of the day, we must recognize when a relationship is no longer serving us and have the courage to let go for the greater good. As Dr. Thema Bryant says, "Leaving a relationship is not an act of hate but of love for yourself" (Bryant, 2022).

Healing from past heartbreak is necessary for love to flourish. The Gottman Institute's research on relationship stability and healthy communication patterns highlights that unhealed emotional wounds from past relationships often show up in new connections (Gottman, 2017). If past love has left you doubting your worth, it's time to rewrite that narrative. Love should never feel like a battlefield. Nurturing our well-being is not frivolous, and it is essential for my wholeness. Part of healing is refusing to let past pain define your future joy, sis. The journey toward love begins within. It's about healing those wounds, setting healthy boundaries, and creating space for love that is kind, supportive, and nurturing.

Is it in Your Heart or Head, Friend?

Love is more than an emotional experience; it is a chemical symphony that plays out in our brains, shaping the way we connect with others. We're about to geek out a little bit with all the science talk, but stay with me. Whether it's the bonds we share with friends, family, or romantic partners, science shows us that love involves fascinating biochemical reactions that deepen our connections and enrich our lives. Far from being abstract, these profound feelings of affection, trust, and happiness are anchored in the release of specific neurotransmitters and hormones that affect our bodies and minds.

A key player in the chemistry of love is oxytocin, often called the "love hormone." According to research, oxytocin is released during intimate moments such as hugging, kissing, and even engaging in deep, heartfelt conversations (Carter, 2014). This hormone acts as a powerful catalyst for social bonding, promoting feelings of closeness and connection between individuals. Oxytocin helps strengthen emotional ties, fostering trust and empathy, essential elements in nurturing healthy relationships. Studies have shown that oxytocin not only increases feelings of love but also reduces stress, making it an essential part of emotional regulation and well-being (MacDonald & MacDonald, 2010).

Alongside oxytocin, other neurotransmitters such as dopamine and serotonin join the love symphony, each contributing its own unique impact. Dopamine, often referred to as the "pleasure hormone," plays a crucial role in the reward system of the brain. It amplifies the joy we experience when we are with those we love, reinforcing the behaviors that make us feel good (Berridge & Robinson, 2003). Dopamine strengthens our desire to nurture and cherish those relationships, pushing us to seek out positive interactions. Serotonin, another key player, contributes to our feelings of emotional well-being, contentment, and calm. Higher levels of serotonin are associated with improved mood and emotional stability, which are vital for sustaining lasting bonds in relationships (Young, 2007).

Understanding these neurochemical reactions can help us appreciate just how much our bodies are involved in our relationships. These hormones and neurotransmitters show that love is not only a feeling but a complex, bodily experience that we can cultivate. Our brain's chemistry works in tandem with our actions, so what we choose to give and receive impacts our neurological well-being.

But love doesn't begin with someone else; it begins with you. The 5 Love Languages by Dr. Gary Chapman is a key resource for understanding how love works on a personal level (Chapman, 1992). Chapman's framework teaches us that everyone expresses and receives love in unique ways, and recognizing this can be transformative for self-love and building meaningful relationships. Whether it's words of affirmation, quality time, acts of service, receiving gifts, or physical touch, knowing your love language is crucial in ensuring you're meeting your own emotional needs. If you crave words of affirmation, start by speaking kindly to yourself…or, you know, let the Ebony Notes app do the heavy lifting for you. If quality time is your love language, make room for solitude and reflection. Loving yourself in your own love language sets the tone for how you allow others to treat you, fostering relationships that align with your authentic needs.

Love is also rooted in community; the friendships, family bonds, and sisterhoods that sustain us. In the works of Toni Morrison, love transcends romantic relationships and becomes a powerful force that defines one's identity. Morrison's novels emphasize that love is grounded in self-worth and in knowing who you are outside of who loves you. In communities, love is found in shared laughter, sisterhood, and mutual support. As Morrison beautifully articulates in *Beloved*, love can both nurture and challenge us, pushing us to grow and evolve (Morrison, 1987). When we cultivate these relationships, we actively build spaces of love, respect, and mutual care.

The neuroscience of love underscores just how profound our experiences of affection and trust can be as we navigate the various forms of love—romantic, familial, platonic, and self-love—our brains orchestrate a symphony of chemical reactions that deepen our emotional bonds. These connections have tangible effects on our physical and mental health, demonstrating the profound impact love has on our overall well-being. Research shows that social support, rooted in love and connection, is linked to better mental health outcomes, lower stress, and increased longevity (Uchino, 2006).

Understanding the role of these neurotransmitters and hormones not only sheds light on the science behind our emotions but also reinforces the importance of love in our lives. The power of love is not merely metaphorical. It is backed by science, showing us that love, in all its forms, is essential to our happiness and overall health.

Vulnerability and Boundaries: The Heart of True Love

Let's talk about vulnerability and boundaries for a minute, sis. These two are at the core of any healthy relationship, whether it's with ourselves or with others. The powerful work of Dr. Brené Brown reminds us that vulnerability is not a weakness but rather a source of strength. It takes courage to open ourselves up to love, to trust, and to allow others to see us as we truly are. In her book Daring Greatly, Brown explains that vulnerability is the birthplace of love, belonging, creativity, and joy (Brown, 2012). Vulnerability isn't about letting people walk all over you. It's about being honest with yourself, showing up authentically, and allowing yourself to experience the depth of connection that love can bring. When we're vulnerable, we create space for real, meaningful connections with others. But the gag is: vulnerability and boundaries go hand in hand.

Setting healthy boundaries is not just a nice idea; it's essential for our emotional well-being. Without boundaries, we risk overextending ourselves, losing touch with our needs, and, ultimately, feeling burnt out and depleted. Dr. Brown emphasizes that boundaries are not just about saying "no" to others; they are about saying "yes" to ourselves. Boundaries protect our emotional energy, helping us maintain our sense of self and prioritize our well-being (Brown, 2012). When we set healthy boundaries, we send a clear message to ourselves and to others that we are worthy of respect, love, and care. We acknowledge that our needs matter and that our peace is a priority. Periodt.

In relationships, whether with family, friends, or romantic partners, setting boundaries is an act of love. It's how we protect our hearts and our souls while still being able to give love freely. When we don't set boundaries, we allow ourselves to become overwhelmed, undervalued, or taken for granted. But when we establish and maintain boundaries, we create a foundation for love that is nurturing, reciprocal, and respectful. Boundaries allow us to love ourselves first so that we can love others more fully. As you navigate your journey toward healing and self-love, remember that healthy boundaries are one of the most important tools you can use to protect your heart, your energy, and your peace.

Remember, setting boundaries doesn't mean we're closing ourselves off or being selfish. It means we are prioritizing our well-being, which, in turn, enables us to show up more fully for the people and causes that matter most to us. Healthy boundaries are not about creating walls; they are about building safe, sacred spaces where love can grow, flourish, and thrive.

Taking Action

- o **Take Inventory of Your Relationships:**
  - o Set aside dedicated time to reflect on the various relationships in your life, including romantic, platonic, familial, and professional relationships.
  - o Create a list or journal entry categorizing each relationship and noting key aspects such as level of closeness, communication patterns, and overall satisfaction.
- o **Assess the Quality of Your Relationships:**
  - o Evaluate each relationship on your list based on factors such as trust, respect, support, and mutual understanding.

- Consider how each relationship makes you feel and whether it contributes positively to your well-being and sense of fulfillment.

- **Identify Strengths and Areas for Improvement:**
  - Acknowledge and celebrate the strengths and positive aspects of your relationships, such as shared values, meaningful connections, and mutual support.
  - Be honest with yourself about any areas where your relationships may be lacking or could benefit from improvement, such as communication challenges, unresolved conflicts, or unmet needs.

- **Reflect on Boundaries and Expectations:**
  - Consider the boundaries you have established in your relationships and whether they are being respected and honored by both parties.
  - Reflect on your expectations for each relationship and whether they align with the reality of the relationship dynamics and interactions.

- **Recognize Signs of Healthy and Unhealthy Relationships:**
  - Educate yourself on the characteristics of healthy, fulfilling relationships, such as mutual respect, effective communication, trust, and support.

- o Be aware of common signs of unhealthy or toxic relationships, such as manipulation, control, lack of boundaries, and emotional or physical abuse.

- o **Communicate Openly and Honestly:**
  - o Practice open and honest communication with your loved ones, expressing your thoughts, feelings, and needs respectfully and assertively.
  - o Encourage your loved ones to do the same, creating a safe and supportive environment for open dialogue and constructive conversations.

- o **Set Goals for Relationship Growth:**
  - o Based on your relationship inventory and assessment, set specific goals for improving the quality and dynamics of your relationships.
  - o Identify actionable steps you can take to work towards these goals, such as initiating difficult conversations, seeking support from a therapist or counselor, or setting aside dedicated quality time with loved ones.

- o **Seek Support and Guidance:**
  - o If you identify areas of concern or struggle in your relationships, consider seeking support and guidance from trusted friends, family members, or professionals.

- o Reach out to a therapist, counselor, or support group specializing in relationships and interpersonal dynamics for personalized guidance and assistance.
- o **Practice Self-Reflection and Self-Care:**
  - o Take time for regular self-reflection to assess your own thoughts, feelings, and behaviors in your relationships and identify areas where you can grow and improve.
  - o Prioritize self-care practices that nurture your mental, emotional, and physical well-being, allowing you to show up as your best self in your relationships.
- o **Celebrate Healthy Relationships:**
  - o Celebrate and express gratitude for the healthy, positive relationships in your life that bring joy, fulfillment, and support.
  - o Show appreciation for your loved ones and celebrate the strengths and unique qualities that make your relationships special.

Here are ten affirmations to help you cultivate love in your life:

1. I am worthy of love and affection.
2. I attract healthy, loving relationships into my life.
3. I am capable of giving and receiving love.
4. I choose partners who respect and honor me.

5. I am deserving of a partner who supports and uplifts me.
6. I am open to giving and receiving love in all its forms.
7. I trust in my ability to navigate relationships with grace and wisdom.
8. I release all fear and insecurities around love and relationships.
9. I am grateful for the love and support in my life.
10. I choose love over fear in all aspects of my life.

In conclusion, love is a powerful force that can bring immense joy and fulfillment to our lives. But it's important to recognize and appreciate all the forms of love in our lives, understand what healthy love looks like, and prioritize our own well-being in our relationships. We deserve the love that is kind, patient, and understanding, and it starts with affirming our own worthiness of love.

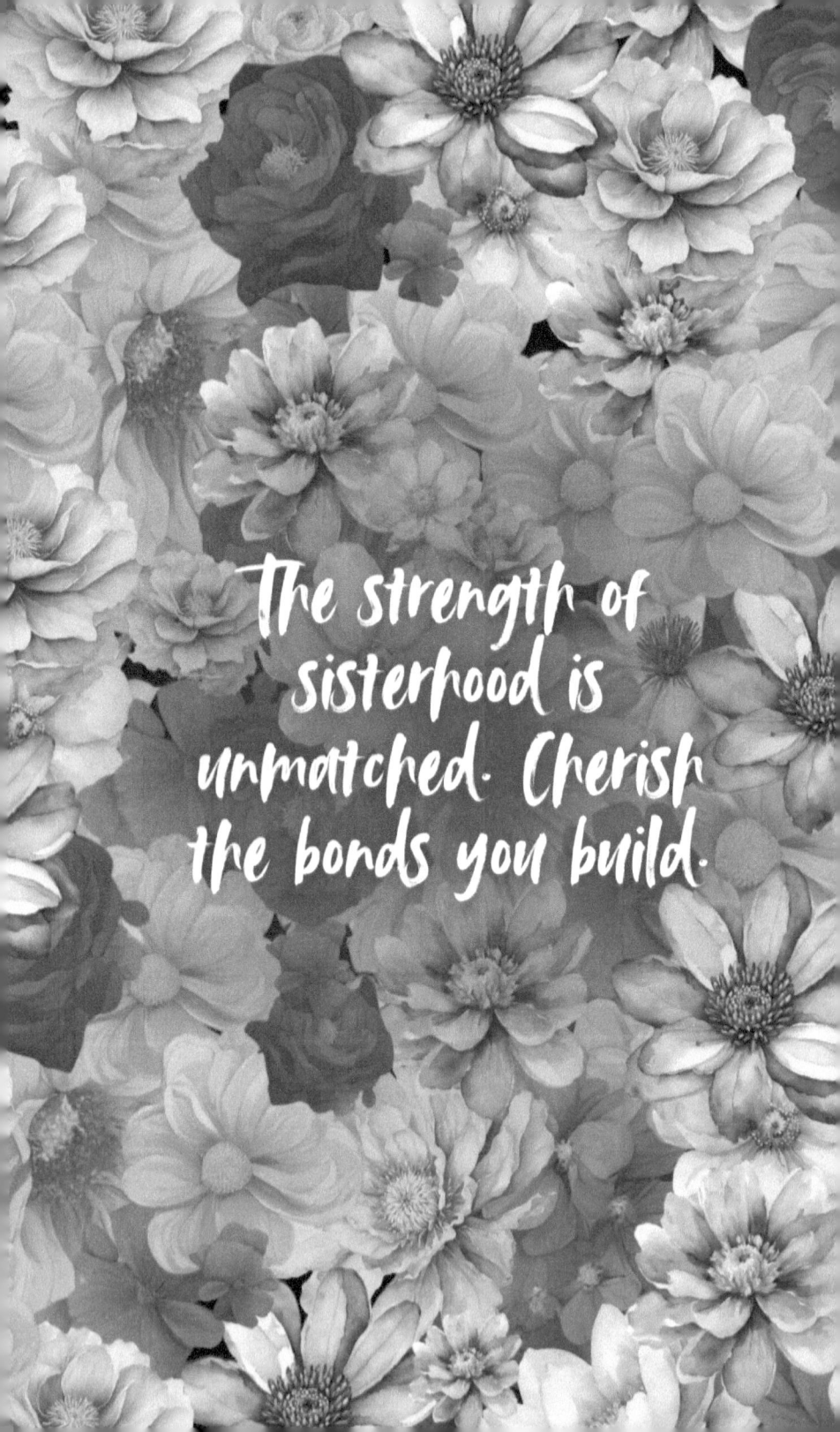

4

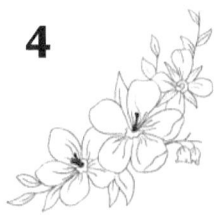

What About Your Friends?

Sis,

Friendship, like love, comes in many forms. Each of us has a unique circle of friends, each playing a different role in our lives. There's the friend who fills our days with laughter, bringing joy and lightness to even the darkest moments. There's the friend with whom we have deep, meaningful conversations, sharing our hopes, fears, and dreams. And then there's the friend who serves as our protector, helping us safeguard our energy and boundaries, ensuring that we prioritize self-care and well-being.

I've personally only rocked within a small circle. Thinking back over the years, in elementary I had 3-4 friends, there was up to 5 by middle school, and for high school through college, I'd say that I was close to 8 people. As an adult, I have about 5 solid friends in my life, if we don't count Mr. Welch.

I've recently learned about having a personal advisory board——a group of friends who serve as our trusted confidants, advisors, and cheerleaders. These are the people we turn to for guidance, encouragement, and honest feedback. They are our sounding board, our shoulder to lean on, and our source of strength when times get tough.

As you reflect on the incredible friendships in your life, cherish these bonds and nurture them with love and gratitude. Remember that you are never alone on this journey. You can create sisterhoods that are unbreakable, resilient, and truly life-affirming.

With all my love and warmest wishes,

Sisterhood

Friendships form the bedrock of our emotional well-being, offering us not just joy but also resilience in the face of life's challenges. For Black women, sisterhood becomes even more essential; it's the sanctuary where we find support and understanding, a place where we can be unapologetically ourselves without fear of judgment. I'll give 2 snaps to that.

Research shows that social support is one of the strongest predictors of mental and emotional health. In *Platonic* by Dr. Marisa G. Franco (2022), we learn that friendship isn't just for companionship; it's an important part of shaping our sense of identity, confidence, and even our longevity. Franco emphasizes that friendship is a balm for life's wounds, providing us with the emotional scaffolding we need to thrive, especially when facing societal pressures unique to Black women.

There are different types of friendships that we may encounter throughout our lives, from childhood friends to work colleagues to online communities. Each type of friendship can bring its own unique benefits and challenges, and it's important to recognize and appreciate the different types of friendships in our lives.

Sisterhood is rooted in shared experiences and collective determinedness. For us, it's a powerful source of healing and solidarity sprinkled with a bit of empowerment. These friendships are more than just social connections; they are spaces of refuge where we can discuss the intersectional challenges we face, from racial injustice to gender bias and everything in between. As author Audre Lorde put it, "Without community, there is no liberation."

Not all friendships are the same, and each one serves a different role in our lives. In *Frientimacy*, Shasta Nelson explains that meaningful friendships are built on three pillars: positivity, consistency, and vulnerability. Some friends bring laughter, others offer deep conversations, and some act as fierce protectors of our peace. A true friendship is not just about history; it's about mutual support and emotional nourishment (Nelson, 2021).

The importance of sisterhood cannot be overstated. It's the kind of friendship where you can laugh until your belly hurts but also cry without any shame. These are the women who show up for you, not just when it's convenient, but especially when life knocks you down. The power of sisterhood lies not just in shared joy but also in mutual vulnerability, compassion, and emotional nourishment.

But it's important to note that not all friendships are created equal. While some friends bring light and joy, others may drain us emotionally, leaving us feeling less than whole. Acknowledging toxic friendships is a vital part of self-love and growth. As Brené Brown teaches us, vulnerability is essential in true connection, but it must be met with respect and trust. Friendships that continually leave us feeling depleted or misunderstood may need reevaluation. Setting clear boundaries and knowing when to walk away is an act of self-preservation, a key step toward maintaining your emotional balance.

In a world that often undervalues Black women, sisterhood and the strength of our friendships can serve as a collective source of empowerment. These friendships are sacred; the women in your circle help anchor you, providing you with the space to be your full self and flaws, all while lifting each other up. As you reflect on the friends in your life, consider whether they are helping you to grow, holding space for your healing, and allowing you to shine unapologetically.

Let's Build Unbreakable Bonds

There's a well-known saying: "You are the sum of the five people you spend the most time with." The friendships you nurture today will shape your growth and guide your future.

Seek out friends who uplift, support, and challenge you in all the right ways. And when you find those friends, hold them close, because Black sisterhood is something worth protecting and celebrating.

As Dr. Joy Harden Bradford explores in *Sisterhood Heals: The Transformative Power of Black Women's Friendships* (2021), the relationships between Black women are vital sources of healing and empowerment. Dr. Joy's research highlights that the deep bonds formed in sisterhood are not only supportive— they are transformative. These friendships help Black women process trauma, create a safe space for vulnerability, and offer the type of healing that only another Black woman can provide. In a world that often disregards our needs, Black sisterhood becomes a sanctuary where we can laugh, cry, and grow together.

Finding your tribe of supportive and like-minded friends can be a powerful experience that can help you navigate the challenges of life with greater ease. It's important to seek out friendships with people who share your values, interests, and experiences. This can involve attending events or groups that align with your interests or joining online communities that cater to your needs. To build your circle of unbreakable bonds, consider joining the Ebony Notes Wellness Community, a space dedicated to supporting Black women, or explore the curated list of other online and offline communities in the resources section to find your tribe.

Opposites Attract

In addition to the powerful bonds we share with our female friends, let's not overlook the significance of friendships with males, friend. These relationships offer a unique perspective, providing insight into the male experience while fostering mutual understanding and support. Society often emphasizes differences between genders, but these friendships remind us of our shared humanity, transcending stereotypes and breaking down the barriers that separate us.

Friendships with males bring diversity to our social circles, enriching our lives with varied perspectives and experiences. They offer companionship, laughter, and a shoulder to lean on during challenging times. But what truly makes these friendships special is the opportunity to learn from one another, bridging the gap between genders while fostering empathy and compassion.

Males often offer a different kind of emotional support that can complement the nurturing, emotionally rich support we often receive from female friends. These relationships are frequently characterized by straightforwardness and practical advice. Males tend to approach problem-solving from a pragmatic angle, offering solutions or actionable guidance. This is particularly beneficial for those of us navigating life's challenges, as it brings a refreshing perspective and sometimes a much-needed reality check.

These friendships also provide a safe space for honest communication and vulnerability, allowing us to express ourselves freely without fear of judgment. We can openly discuss things like career challenges, relationships, and mental well-being. Males in these relationships are often less likely to make us feel like we are "too much" for expressing our emotions, fostering an environment of understanding where we can truly be ourselves.

Importantly, these connections challenge us to see beyond gender roles and expectations. Instead of limiting ourselves to traditional views of what friendships between men and women should look like, we can embrace each other as individuals with unique strengths, weaknesses, and experiences. In doing so, we celebrate the richness that comes from diverse social circles. Gender should never be a barrier to meaningful connection, and it is this diversity in our friendships that contributes to our growth as individuals.

Psychologist Dr. Deborah Tannen discusses in *You Just Don't Understand* that men and women often communicate differently, but those differences don't diminish the value of the connection. Instead, they allow for an exchange of perspectives that helps both genders grow. In fact, having diverse friendships—across gender lines—can deepen our emotional intelligence, expand our understanding of others, and ultimately improve our relationship-building skills.

These friendships also contribute significantly to our well-being. A 2018 study published in *Psychological Science* found that positive male friendships are associated with lower levels of depression and anxiety. These friendships provide us with camaraderie and emotional validation, giving us the confidence to thrive both personally and professionally.

As we celebrate the diverse friendships in our lives, let us appreciate the unique bond we share with our male friends. They provide us with more than just companionship; they enrich our lives with varied insights, emotional support, and mutual respect. Regardless of gender, these connections contribute to our holistic well-being, making us feel supported, understood, and empowered. Let's cherish the meaningful relationships that make us whole, whether they are with women, men, or anyone who brings value into our lives.

Season, Reason, or Lifetime

As we navigate the complexities of friendships, it's important to recognize that some connections are meant to be temporary, serving a specific purpose or season in our lives. Some friendships come into our lives to teach us something, give us companionship during a particular chapter, or guide us through a specific challenge. In her book *Platonic*, Dr. Marisa G. Franco reminds us that it's natural for friendships to evolve as we do. She writes, "Friendships should help you evolve into the best version of yourself, not hold you back" (Franco, 2022). It's easy to feel obligated to hold onto every relationship that has ever been important to us, but sometimes, allowing certain friendships to run their course creates the space we need to grow.

Black sisterhood, from the strength and unity displayed in the Civil Rights Movement to the modern-day activism we see, has always been a profound source of collective strength. But even these powerful bonds evolve over time. Sisterhood is a living entity; one that shifts and changes, reflecting the unique needs and circumstances of each phase of our lives. Whether it's due to personal growth, shifts in life direction, or differing values, the ebb and flow of relationships don't diminish their significance.

Just like the seasons change, so do our friendships. This is perfectly okay. As we continue on our journeys of self-discovery and growth, our circle of friends may shift accordingly. Sometimes, it can feel bittersweet to acknowledge when friendships no longer serve us or align with our values and aspirations. But the truth is, we evolve, and so must the people who walk alongside us. In the words of Maya Angelou, "When people show you who they are, believe them the first time." This applies to friendships as well; we must accept when relationships no longer align with who we are becoming.

It's important to honor the friendships that serve us now while also making peace with those who have run their course. It's also essential to recognize that growth often comes from the courage to let go. When friendships no longer offer the support, love, and trust you need, it's okay to move on. As you make room for the right people, you create space for new, uplifting relationships that will reflect the person you're becoming.

By understanding that friendships, like seasons, come and go, we can begin to celebrate the role each person played in our lives and release them with love. Trust that new connections and opportunities for growth will emerge as you evolve. The season, reason, or lifetime of a friendship may be brief or long, but each one plays an important part in shaping who you are and who you are becoming.

a Note from LaDonna

Alright, sister friend, let's talk real talk. Are you holding it down in the friendship department?

First things first, make sure you are doing all the things that you expect from your circle. Friendship isn't just about the fun times, it's about being there through the thick and thin, the highs and lows, the Netflix marathons, and the ugly cries. Evaluate yourself and determine if you may need to step your game up.

Being a good friend isn't all serious business either. Sometimes, it's about the little things, like sending a funny meme or just checking in. It's about knowing when to listen, when to laugh, and when to pass the tissues.

So, ask yourself, sis: Do you need to level up in the friendship department? What we put out in the world is just as important as what we expect to receive.

Taking Action

o **Conduct a Friendship Inventory:** Take some time to evaluate your current friendships and assess whether they align with your values, aspirations, and personal growth journey. Consider the level of support, respect, and positivity each friendship brings into your life.

o **Identify Common Interests:** Explore your interests, hobbies, and passions, and seek out opportunities to connect with individuals who share similar interests. Join clubs, groups, or organizations centered around activities you enjoy, and use these spaces to meet like-minded individuals and forge new friendships.

o **Expand Your Social Network:** Expand your social network by challenging yourself to step out of your comfort zone. Attend social events, workshops, or community gatherings, and be open to meeting new people and engaging in meaningful conversations. Seize opportunities to connect with individuals who resonate with you on a personal or professional level, and embrace the chance to cultivate diverse friendships outside of your usual social circles.

o **Cultivate Meaningful Connections:** Invest time and effort in nurturing meaningful connections with individuals who share your interests, values, and goals. Focus on building authentic, supportive relationships based on mutual trust, respect, and shared experiences.

o **Practice Active Listening:** Enhance your communication skills and deepen your connections with others by practicing active listening. Make a conscious effort to listen attentively, empathize with others' perspectives, and validate their feelings and experiences.

o **Be Open-Minded:** Approach new friendships with an open mind and a willingness to embrace diversity and difference. Be receptive to learning from others, exploring new perspectives, and celebrating the unique qualities and backgrounds that each individual brings to the table.

o **Attend Social Gatherings:** Take advantage of social gatherings, community events, or networking opportunities to meet new people and expand your social network. Engage in meaningful conversations, exchange contact information, and follow up with potential new friends to nurture budding friendships.

o **Nurture Existing Friendships**: Invest time and effort in nurturing existing friendships by staying connected, reaching out regularly, and making meaningful gestures to show appreciation and support for your friends. Schedule regular catch-ups, outings, or virtual hangouts to maintain strong connections and deepen your bonds over time.

o **Be Open to Change:** Embrace the natural evolution of friendships and be open to change as your social circle grows and evolves over time. Recognize that friendships may ebb and flow, and be willing to adapt to shifting dynamics and priorities while prioritizing relationships that bring positivity, fulfillment, and mutual support into your life.

Drake may have said, "No New Friends," but let's be real, sis—sometimes we have to revisit those words and challenge them a little. Sure, it sounds cool at the moment, especially when you've been burned or disappointed by people you thought had your back. But before you hold onto that mantra too tightly, reread points 6 and 9, and consider the possibility that new friendships might just be the answer you need.

God places people in our lives for a reason, a season, or a lifetime. Not everyone is meant to stay, but everyone has a purpose in our journey. We can't always know what that purpose is at first glance, but often, the new people who come into our lives hold lessons, opportunities, and perspectives we couldn't have predicted. Sometimes, they're meant to walk with us through a chapter we're not quite ready for on our own, and other times, they open doors that we didn't even know were closed.

You never really know what a new friendship might bring. It could be someone who introduces you to a new opportunity, challenges you to think differently, or becomes the very person who helps you step into a new chapter of your life. Just like in nature, sometimes the right new connection is the one that blooms where you've planted new seeds. Maybe it's a bond that will blossom into something deep, or maybe it's one that's only meant to be in your life for a short time. But don't let that deter you from being open to the people God places in your path.

Every new connection is an invitation—to expand, to grow, and to learn something new about yourself. So, instead of blocking those who could bring you joy, growth, or even a fresh perspective, be open to the possibility that this new friend might be the one to help you break through to the next level of your life.

Here are ten affirmations for Black women's friendships:

1. I am deserving of genuine and supportive friendships.
2. I am grateful for the strong sisterhood of women in my life.
3. I am capable of being a good friend to others.
4. I attract positive and uplifting friendships into my life.
5. I am open to making new friendships that align with my values and interests.
6. I am a valuable and appreciated member of my friend group.
7. I prioritize healthy boundaries in my friendships to maintain my well-being.
8. I communicate openly and honestly with my friends to strengthen our relationships.
9. I make time for my friendships and prioritize nurturing these connections.

10. I am grateful for the diversity of experiences and perspectives that my friendships bring into my life.

To wrap this up, friendships are a vital part of our lives, bringing us joy, laughter, and support. As Black women, cultivating a strong sisterhood is essential for navigating the unique challenges we face. We deserve friendships that align with our values, honor our boundaries, and uplift us—because we are worthy of connections that empower and nourish us.

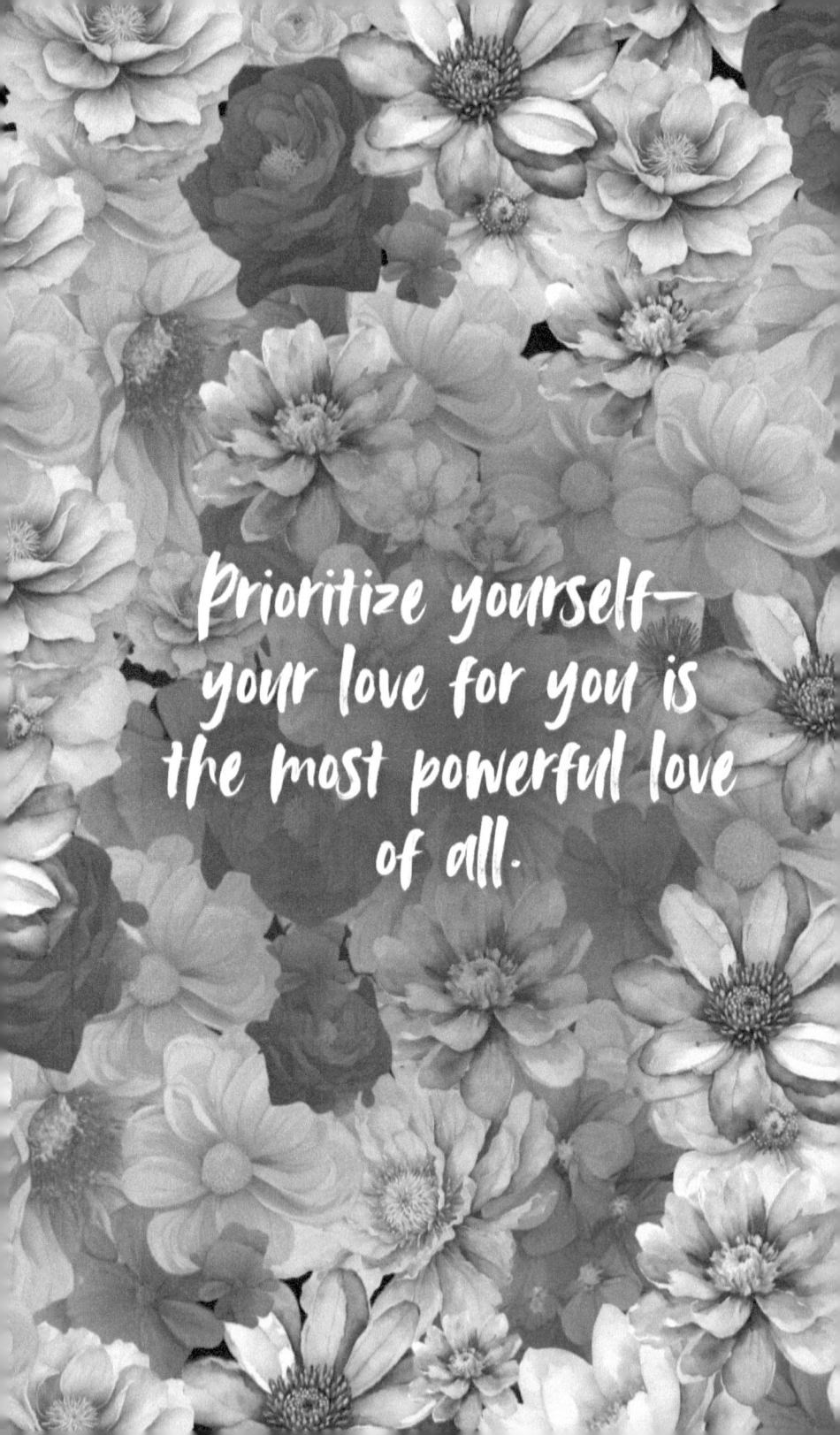

Prioritize yourself—
your love for you is
the most powerful love
of all.

5

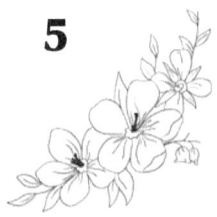

Self—love is Not Selfish

To My Fellow Goddess,

In exploring the journey of self-love, it's essential to recognize its transformative power, a power that extends far beyond ourselves and touches every aspect of our lives. Let's delve into the profound impact self-love has on our relationships with others, highlighting the importance of loving oneself to love others genuinely.

You, cherished sister, are deserving of boundless love and acceptance. When you nurture a deep sense of love and compassion within yourself, you're better equipped to extend that same love to those around you. Just as tending to a garden yields abundant blossoms, nurturing self-love allows your capacity for sharing love and kindness with others to flourish.

Moreover, self-love is integral to your well-being and happiness. It's about honoring your worthiness, celebrating your uniqueness, and embracing your journey with compassion and grace. By practicing self-love, you fortify your resilience, deepen your empathy, and create space for meaningful connections.

Self-love is Not Selfish

It's important to understand that self-love isn't selfish; it's an act of preserving your peace and care. By setting healthy boundaries, prioritizing your needs, and acknowledging your inherent value as an individual, you affirm your worthiness of love and respect, from both others and yourself

So, I invite you to embark on this journey of self-love with an open heart and a spirit of compassion. Embrace every facet of who you are, forgive yourself for past shortcomings, and bask in the glow of your inherent worthiness. As you cultivate self-love, may you find that your capacity for authentic connection and love expands, enriching your life and the lives of those around you.

Keep Lovin' Yourself,

A Journey, Not a Destination

I've mentioned this before and will do so again, Black women have historically been expected to be strong for everyone else, often at the expense of their own well-being. Toni Morrison explored this in Beloved, where the weight of generational trauma shapes how Black women view themselves. This is why self-love isn't just personal, it's deeply connected to history. Beyoncé's Cozy serves as a modern-day reminder that Black women deserve to be comfortable in their skin, fully embracing who they are without apology. She sang, "I'm comfortable in my skin, cozy with who I am." And I felt that! Beyoncé's lyrics remind us that true self-love involves embracing our authenticity despite the external pressures to conform or shrink. It's a radical act to accept and love ourselves as we are fully, and in doing so, we heal generations of hurt and recover our peace.

Self-love is not a luxury, it's a necessity. Dr. Kristin Neff, a leading researcher on self-compassion, explains that self-kindness is crucial for emotional resilience and long-term well-being. When you prioritize yourself, you're not being selfish. You're affirming that you deserve care, peace, and joy. As the late Maya Angelou wisely said, 'You alone are enough. You have nothing to prove to anybody' (Angelou, 2008). In a world that often demands we put everyone else first, choosing ourselves is a revolutionary act.

Self-love is a journey that requires patience, compassion, and courage, especially as Black women facing external pressures that can make it challenging to prioritize our own needs. Cultivating self-love allows us to accept and appreciate ourselves fully, countering the conditioning to prioritize others over ourselves. It's essential for our well-being, enabling us to live happier, healthier, and more fulfilling lives.

Loving yourself fully is crucial not only for your own happiness and well-being but also for nurturing healthy relationships with others. Embracing self-love enables you to love and accept others more readily while establishing healthy boundaries that foster mutual respect and understanding. Recognizing that self-love is not selfish but rather an essential foundation for genuine connection, we realize that by loving and accepting ourselves, we become better equipped to extend love and compassion to others authentically and sustainably. Now, read that again!

Dr. Kristin Neff's research on self-compassion has shown that when we practice self-love, we not only significantly improve our emotional well-being but also increase our ability to support others effectively. Self-compassion allows individuals to embrace their imperfections without shame, an essential practice for Black women who often carry the weight of societal expectations.

The Foundation for Comprehensive Growth

Self-love serves as the foundation for comprehensive growth, nurturing our physical, psychological, and spiritual well-being. Prioritizing self-love encompasses activities that sustain our bodies, such as exercise, healthy eating, and restful sleep, while also nurturing our psychological health through seeking support, managing stress, and engaging in self-reflection. It's all interconnected, sis. Self-love facilitates spiritual growth by fostering a connection with our higher self and purpose, promoting alignment with our values.

Incorporating self-love enhances our psychological and spiritual evolution. By embracing all facets of ourselves, including our imperfections and missteps, we foster inner peace and acceptance. This liberation empowers us to transcend feelings of shame, guilt, or self-doubt that may impede our progress. Through nurturing our inner wisdom and intuition, we gain the clarity needed to make choices that resonate with our values and fulfill our purpose.

Cultivating self-love fuels growth across every dimension of our existence, fostering freedom, confidence, and empowerment as cornerstones of personal development. By prioritizing our well-being and establishing healthy boundaries, we forge a foundation of safety and stability that emboldens us to pursue our aspirations. Furthermore, investing in our physical health amplifies our vitality and energy, empowering us to engage in all aspects of life fully. Now that's a word!

Research from Harvard Medical School has shown that practicing self-compassion positively impacts physical health by reducing stress and boosting immune function. Similarly, investing in one's mental and physical health through self-love practices helps individuals cultivate self-dependence and long-term wellness.

Rest is Essential

Rest is an essential part of self-love. The Nap Ministry, founded by Tricia Hersey, challenges the idea that overworking is a badge of honor, especially for Black women. Rest is not laziness; it's a form of resistance against systems that thrive on our exhaustion. If you're constantly running on empty, you're not able to show up as your best self.

Prioritizing rest isn't just self-care; it's reclaiming your right to be well.

Tricia Hersey's work emphasizes the importance of rest as a form of resistance, particularly for Black women who are disproportionately affected by burnout and overwork. Hersey's advocacy for rest as resistance helps Black women regain their agency and demand the space to recover and rejuvenate.

Through self-love, we honor our boundaries and embrace what nourishes our souls without apology. We confidently decline what doesn't serve us and enthusiastically seize opportunities that bring us joy and fulfillment. With self-love as our guide, we take deliberate action to shape the life we desire, whether it involves pursuing a new career, ending toxic relationships, or prioritizing our mental well-being.

When you love yourself, you set the tone for how others treat you. In Self-Compassion, Dr. Neff highlights that people with high self-worth naturally attract healthier relationships because they don't tolerate mistreatment or settle for less. Self-love isn't just about what you think of yourself—it influences the standards you uphold in every aspect of your life, from your relationships to your career.

You are worthy of love, care, and happiness; no validation is needed. The world may tell us otherwise, but Black women have always created spaces for self-affirmation. From Maya Angelou's Phenomenal Woman to the self-love anthems of Lizzo, there's proof all around us that our worth is not up for debate. The more we believe in our own values, the less we seek external validation to define us.

a Note from LaDonna

This is the Super Bowl of this book, y'all. Self-love is the foundation. I don't think you 'heard' me. Without self-love, everything else is irrelevant.

Let's be radical with our self-love. What does that mean? It means tearing down the walls of self-doubt and insecurity, and instead, embracing ourselves fully and unapologetically.

Rejecting societal standards of beauty and worth and defining our own value on our own terms.

Prioritizing our own well-being and happiness above all else, unafraid to set boundaries and say no when necessary.

Radical self-love is about honoring our truths, embracing our flaws, and celebrating our unique identities. It's a revolutionary act in a world that often tells us we're not enough.

Taking Action

o **Embrace Your Authenticity:** Celebrate your unique identity as a Black woman and embrace all aspects of yourself, including your culture, heritage, and individuality. Recognize that your authenticity is your greatest strength, and honor your true self without apology or compromise.

o **Practice Radical Self-Acceptance:** Release the need for perfection and embrace yourself exactly as you are, flaws and all. Practice radical self-acceptance by acknowledging and embracing every part of yourself, including your imperfections, insecurities, and vulnerabilities.

o **Set Boundaries and Prioritize Your Needs:** Honor your own needs and well-being by setting clear boundaries with others and prioritizing self-care. Learn to say no without guilt or explanation and advocate for yourself in all areas of your life, including relationships, work, and personal pursuits.

o **Cultivate Self-Compassion:** Treat yourself with the same kindness, compassion, and understanding that you would offer to a cherished friend or loved one. Practice self-compassion by acknowledging your struggles and challenges with empathy and gentleness, and offer yourself words of encouragement and support.

o **Nourish Your Mind, Body, and Soul:** Prioritize your physical, emotional, and spiritual well-being by engaging in activities that nourish and replenish your mind, body, and soul. Dedicate time each day, even if it's just 10 minutes, to activities that bring you joy, peace, and fulfillment, whether it's journaling, meditating, dancing, or spending time in nature.

o **Surround Yourself with Positive Influences:** Consider this for everything that you consume, from music, your social feed, what you read, places you visit, etc. Curate your inner circle to include people who uplift, inspire, and support you on your journey of self-love and self-discovery. Surround yourself with positive influences who celebrate your strengths, encourage your growth, and honor your worth as a Black woman. Are these things, experiences, or people building you up are tearing you down?

o **Challenge Negative Self-Talk:** Become aware of the negative self-talk and internalized beliefs that undermine your self-worth and replace them with affirming, empowering thoughts and beliefs. Challenge the inner critic with self-affirming statements that reinforce your value, worthiness, and beauty.

o **Practice Gratitude and Appreciation:** Cultivate an attitude of gratitude by regularly expressing appreciation for yourself, your experiences, and the blessings in your life. Take time each day to reflect on the things you're grateful for and acknowledge the abundance that surrounds you, fostering a sense of contentment and fulfillment.

o **Invest in Your Personal Growth:** Commit to lifelong learning and personal development by seeking out opportunities to expand your knowledge, skills, and talents. Invest in your personal growth by taking courses, attending workshops, reading books, and pursuing activities that inspire and challenge you.

o **Celebrate Your Uniqueness:** Embrace your individuality and celebrate the qualities, talents, and strengths that make you uniquely you. Recognize that your uniqueness is a gift to be celebrated and shared with the world, and allow yourself to shine brightly as the beautiful, radiant Black woman that you are. Beyoncé's 'Brown Skin Girl' celebrates the beauty and brilliance of Black women in all shades, reminding us that we were never meant to shrink ourselves. Auntie Tabitha Brown, with her warmth and wisdom, teaches us that authenticity is our superpower—when we show up as our full selves, the world makes room for us.

Here are ten affirmations for Black women's self-love:

1. I am worthy of love and respect, including from myself.
2. I embrace my flaws and imperfections as part of my unique beauty.
3. I prioritize my own needs and well-being without guilt or shame.
4. I am capable of achieving my goals and dreams, and I believe in myself.
5. I am grateful for my body and treat it with love and care.
6. I forgive myself for my mistakes and learn from them.
7. I trust my intuition and make decisions that align with my values and goals.
8. I surround myself with positive and uplifting energy.
9. I celebrate my accomplishments and progress, no matter how small.
10. I love myself unconditionally and completely.

Ultimately, self-love is about honoring and respecting ourselves fully, without apology. When we prioritize our own well-being and happiness, we set a powerful example for others to do the same. We become role models for self-love and empower others to embrace their own worth and value. As the saying goes, "Taking action is the highest form of self-love." So, let's take action to love and accept ourselves fully and inspire others to do the same.

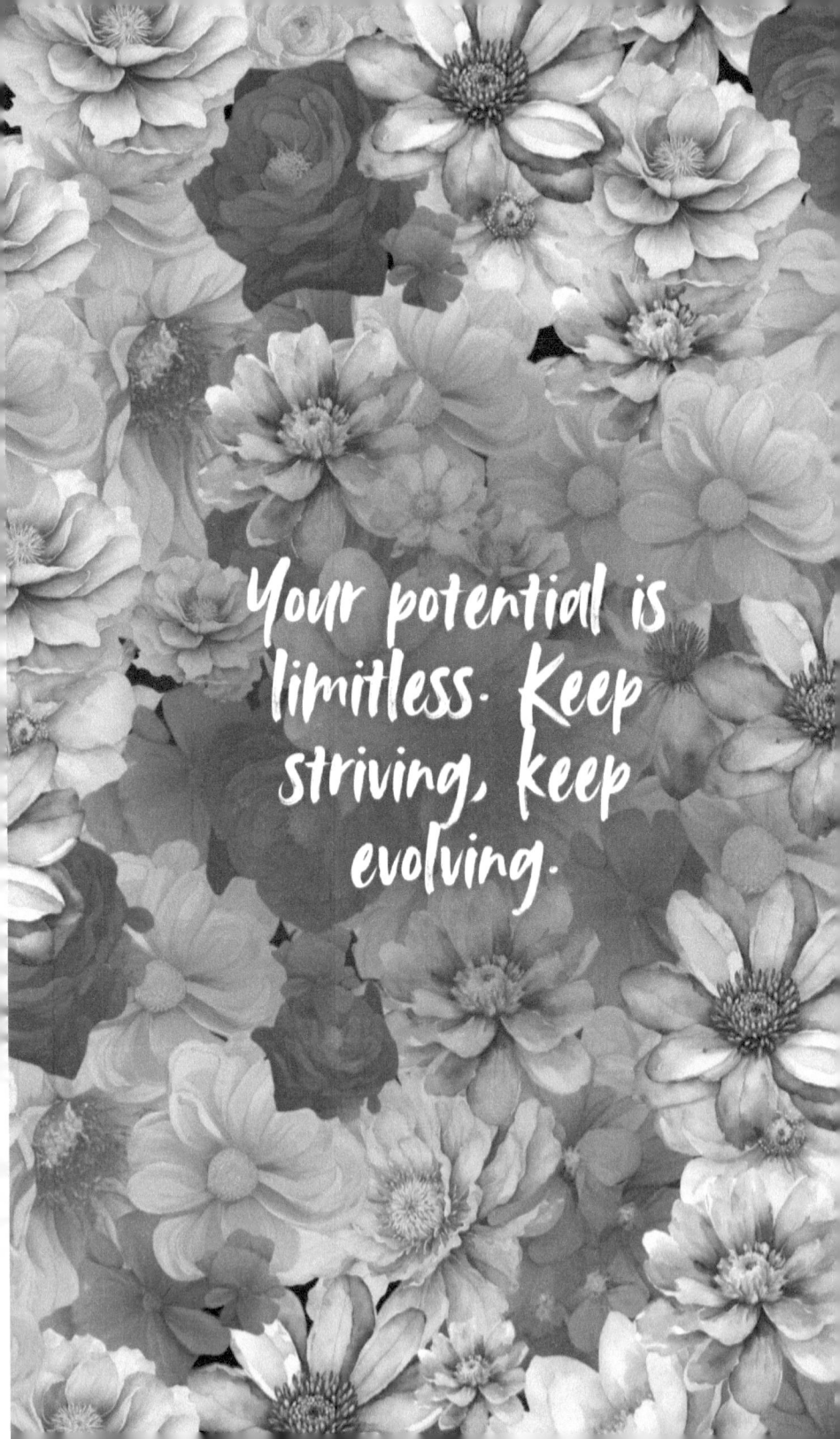

6

Growth for Black Women

Hey Queen,

Contemplating the journey of personal growth fills me with awe and gratitude for the incredible potential that resides within each of us. Let's consider the beauty of growth; the power of evolving, the strength found in stepping out of our comfort zones, and the myriad ways in which we can nurture our growth mindset.

Growth is not just about physical maturation, it's about expanding our minds, our hearts, and our spirits. Embracing change, facing challenges with persistence, and continuously striving to become the best versions of ourselves define this journey. It's a path of self-discovery, self-improvement, and self-realization that knows no bounds.

At the core of growth lies a growth mindset, an unwavering belief in our ability to learn, adapt, and grow from every experience life presents us. Seeing setbacks as opportunities for growth, failures as lessons to be learned, and obstacles as stepping stones to success, we cultivate resilience, perseverance, and a sense of empowerment that propels us forward on our journey.

But growth also requires us to step out of our comfort zones, to embrace discomfort, uncertainty, and vulnerability. It's in these moments of discomfort that we experience the most profound growth, pushing past our limitations and discovering the strength and determination that lie within us.

As we journey through life, we encounter various types of growth: mental growth, social growth, spiritual growth, emotional growth, and physical growth. Each type contributes to our overall development and well-being, enriching our lives in countless ways.

So, my dear, I encourage you to embrace the beauty of growth; to lean into discomfort, cultivate a growth mindset, and celebrate every step forward on your journey. May you continue to evolve, learn, and grow into the magnificent person you are meant to be.

Keep Growing,

Growing Pains

As Black women, we're up against some real challenges that can hinder our personal growth and development. From dealing with systemic oppression, racism, and sexism to facing all kinds of societal expectations and cultural norms that dictate how we should act, look, and feel, it's like we're constantly walking a tightrope. In a world that sometimes feels like it was built for everyone except us, it can feel overwhelming. But you know what? Despite all that, we have to keep pushing forward and never stop growing by prioritizing our personal growth and development continuously.

This struggle is not a new one. Our foremothers like Audre Lorde, Maya Angelou, and bell hooks have paved the way, urging us to keep fighting and to persist in our own healing and empowerment. Bell Hooks reminds us in All About Love that love isn't just about romantic relationships—it's also about self-love, community, and pushing for equality and justice. She writes, "To love well is the most powerful tool for change." In many ways, personal growth, particularly for Black women, becomes a form of resistance to the systems that seek to keep us small.

We're told to conform, to be unyielding at the cost of our own well-being. But, sister, let me tell you, growing pains are real, and they are okay! Growth is uncomfortable. It requires stepping into the unknown, embracing challenges, and pushing past limitations. As Carol Dweck, a psychologist at Stanford University, highlighted in her groundbreaking research on mindset, those who have a "growth mindset"—a belief that abilities and intelligence can be developed—are more likely to succeed, especially when faced with challenges. Her work shows us that growth isn't just about natural talent but about effort, learning, and tenaciousness.

Just imagine how different our experience could be if we were encouraged to see every challenge as an opportunity rather than a setback. Angela Duckworth, in her book Grit, expands on this by pointing out that perseverance and passion, not just talent, are the true markers of success. When you think about it, how many times have we pushed through adversity, whether at work, school or in our personal lives, because we refused to quit? Black women have been doing this for generations, turning our pain into power and finding new paths in the face of seemingly impossible odds.

In this journey, it's important to recognize that growth isn't linear. It isn't about a destination but about the consistent effort to evolve. The challenges we face don't just define us, they refine us. They teach us how strong we really are, and through embracing the process, we gain wisdom and clarity.

So, my dear, never let the obstacles of life deter you. Know that every difficulty you face is contributing to your transformation. Instead of shying away from the growing pains, lean into them. That discomfort? It's what makes us stronger, wiser, and more empowered to thrive.

Mindset is Everything: Adopting a Growth Mindset

Personal growth is like our secret weapon, girl. It's the tool we use to break barriers, achieve our dreams, and become the best version of ourselves. Personal growth refers to the intentional and continuous effort to develop oneself in various areas of life: mental, emotional, spiritual, and even physical. It's about putting in that daily effort to better ourselves, however minuscule the step may seem. And let me tell you, it's a game-changer. Growth isn't just a nice idea; it's an essential part of living a fulfilling life. As Black women, we must strive to grow and evolve continuously, not just for our own benefit but for the generations that will follow.

Growth is not something that just happens; it's something we actively choose. It's a mindset that we have to nurture every day. Embracing a growth mindset means we believe that we can learn, evolve, and improve. It means we're willing to step into new experiences and take on challenges, knowing that every failure is just a lesson in disguise. As Carol Dweck, the psychologist behind the concept of a growth mindset, explains, "The passion for stretching yourself and sticking to it, even (or especially) when it's not going well, is the hallmark of the growth mindset." This mindset is a game-changer, and it's the foundation of everything we do in our personal growth journey.

When you have a growth mindset, you approach the world with an openness to learning and expanding. You stop fearing failure and start seeing it as part of the process. Instead of feeling defeated when things don't go as planned, you take it as an opportunity to reflect, adjust, and improve. Angela Duckworth, in her book Grit, shows us that success doesn't come from talent alone; as previously mentioned, it comes from passion and perseverance, and that's exactly what we need to build within ourselves. Growth isn't linear, but that doesn't mean it's not happening. Every day, we are evolving, learning, and becoming more resilient.

As Black women, we face unique challenges, but we also possess a well of strength and resolve. Our history is filled with examples of women who have overcome incredible obstacles, from Madam C.J. Walker, who built a multi-million-dollar beauty empire despite the odds, to Maya Angelou, whose words continue to inspire generations. These women didn't let setbacks define them; they saw each challenge as an opportunity to grow stronger, wiser, and more powerful. Their mindset was rooted in the belief that growth is a lifelong journey, and they didn't stop until they reached the heights they deserved.

The beauty of a growth mindset is that it can be cultivated. It's not something you're born with; it's something you develop. Each time you face a challenge and push through, you build that mindset. It's about making the decision to grow, even when it's hard. And with that decision comes transformation: mentally, emotionally, and spiritually.

So, my sister, I encourage you to adopt that growth mindset. Embrace every challenge that comes your way with open arms, knowing that you are capable of overcoming it. Understand that every time you fall, you have the strength to get back up. You have everything you need within you to succeed. The world may try to box you in, but with a growth mindset, you are limitless. This is your journey of self-discovery, and every step forward, even if it seems trivial, is a victory.

Stepping Out of the Comfort Zone: Embracing Discomfort

Sis, if we want to grow, we've got to step out of our comfort zones. I know, I know. It sounds easier said than done. But let me tell you, this is where the magic happens. The minute we step out of what feels safe and familiar, we unlock a new realm of possibilities and opportunities for growth. And while it might feel uncomfortable at first, believe me, it's so worth it.

Growth doesn't happen in the comfort zone. It happens when we take risks, face the unknown, and challenge ourselves to do what we never thought possible. As humans, we tend to seek comfort. It's natural. But in staying comfortable, we limit ourselves. We box ourselves in, not allowing ourselves to reach our full potential. True growth, however, lies beyond the known, and it requires a willingness to embrace discomfort. It's like stretching before a workout; you have to push past the initial resistance to reach new levels.

This doesn't mean we need to jump into the deep end immediately, but it does mean we need to start taking small steps outside of the norm. Each step outside that zone builds confidence and capability, helping us unlock new skills, meet new people, and most importantly, discover just how resilient we truly are. So don't shy away from those uncomfortable situations. Whether it's applying for that job that scares you, speaking up when you usually stay quiet, or traveling to a new place solo, these are the experiences that stretch you, that push you, and that help you grow.

Psychologist Carol Dweck, in her book Mindset, explains that people who adopt a growth mindset, those who are willing to step outside their comfort zones, tend to achieve more because they embrace challenges rather than avoid them. It's about seeing failure as a lesson, not a setback. Embracing discomfort is the ultimate sign of growth; it shows you're willing to evolve, adapt, and keep going despite the bumps along the way.

As Black women, we've been conditioned to be resilient, to rise above, and to push through adversity. But sometimes, that adversity comes from the fear of stepping out of our comfort zones. Maybe it's the fear of judgment or rejection. Maybe it's the fear of failure. But what if we flip that narrative? What if we start seeing discomfort not as something to avoid but as an invitation to level up? The more we practice discomfort, the more resilient and confident we become. And that's exactly what we need to continue evolving into the badass women we are meant to be.

It's in those moments of discomfort that we find our strength. It's when we push through the initial fear that we realize just how capable we are. The late Maya Angelou once said, "We may encounter many defeats, but we must not be defeated." Every moment of discomfort is simply a chance to grow stronger, wiser, and more equipped to handle whatever comes our way.

The beauty of stepping outside your comfort zone is that it's not just about reaching new goals; it's about learning who you are along the way. You discover new strengths, new capabilities, and new passions. You begin to realize that you're capable of more than you ever thought possible.

The Power of Community: Growth is Collective

Sis, let's talk about something that is often underestimated in our journeys of personal growth: the power of community. We've all heard the phrase "It takes a village," and that's no different when it comes to personal development. Your growth doesn't just benefit you, and it benefits everyone around you. When you step into your fullest potential, you create opportunities for others to rise too. This is the beauty of collective growth.

Dr. Joy DeGruy, in her groundbreaking work on Post-Traumatic Slave Syndrome, teaches us that healing and empowerment within Black communities are not isolated events; they ripple out, touching every single one of us. The impact of one Black woman's growth can have a profound and lasting effect on generations to come. Whether it's through mentorship, business ventures, or simply by leading with purposefulness and strength, the power of one can catalyze a movement. As we grow, we build stronger communities, and in turn, these communities support and nurture more growth. This is why growth is not just personal; it's collective.

Our personal achievements become the collective's fuel. When one Black woman wins, we all win. Issa Rae, who's built an empire from the ground up, famously said, "I'm rooting for everybody Black." And let me tell you, this mindset speaks volumes. It's a reminder of how important it is to celebrate each other's successes. When we uplift each other, we create a network of support that sustains and empowers us all. This is community at its finest, where success is not a competition but a collective celebration.

Building a supportive community is vital. It's about surrounding yourself with people who inspire you to be better, who push you to go further, and who hold space for your growth. Whether through mentorship, sisterhood, or networking, these connections allow us to rise together, not just as individuals, but as a collective force. Black women, when we unite, we create a space where success is not only possible but also inevitable.

Community is where we share knowledge, resources, and wisdom, and it's in these spaces that we can heal from the collective trauma we've experienced. The healing of one becomes the healing of many. Just look at the history of Black women, whether it was the Civil Rights Movement, Black Lives Matter, or any other movement for social change; the collective strength and wisdom of Black women have always been the driving force behind progress. We lead the way, and when we support one another, our strength multiplies.

By prioritizing the growth of those around us, we unlock the power of collective transformation. Whether through networking or just showing up for each other, the power of community enables us to break down barriers and build paths to success for the next generation.

a Note from LaDonna

For real, let's talk straight facts: Black women are out here killin' it.

I mean, we're holding it down as the most educated and accomplished group, period. Despite all the obstacles thrown our way, we keep hustling, grinding, and shining like the queens we are.

From the boardroom to the classroom, we're making moves and breaking barriers left and right. It's inspiring to see how we're changing the game and leaving our mark on the world.

Our contributions and achievements are invaluable, and our impact on society is profound.

So, let's give props where they're due and show some love to all our Black queens for all that we do!

Types of Personal Growth: Mental, Social, Spiritual, Emotional, and Physical

Personal growth is not a one-size-fits-all approach. We must focus on all aspects of ourselves, our minds, bodies, and spirits, to thrive truly. When we prioritize balanced growth, we ensure that we evolve holistically, addressing each facet of our lives to create a life of fulfillment, purpose, and well-being.

There are several types of personal growth, each contributing uniquely to our overall development. Mental growth is about cultivating our cognitive abilities—our ability to think critically, solve problems, and expand our knowledge. Social growth involves building our communication and interpersonal skills, enhancing our relationships with others, and fostering connections. Spiritual growth is about nourishing our inner self, deepening our connection with a higher power, and aligning with our personal values. Emotional growth focuses on enhancing our emotional intelligence and self-reliance, and physical growth centers on nurturing our health and fitness.

Our mental growth is key, especially in the face of the societal biases and stereotypes that often try to define who we are. Mental growth isn't just about acquiring knowledge—it's about constantly challenging ourselves to think critically and to step outside of our comfort zones. Each time we engage with new concepts, read books, or have deep conversations, we stimulate our minds and break down the mental barriers that limit us.

By developing our mental faculties, we equip ourselves to navigate the world with confidence, creativity, and intelligence. It also helps us to manage the emotional and psychological toll that the external pressures on Black women can bring. Prioritizing mental growth by challenging ourselves through activities like reading, taking courses, or engaging in intellectually stimulating conversations helps us keep our minds sharp and our spirits resilient.

When it comes to social growth, we need to acknowledge the unique challenges Black women face in expressing themselves authentically due to societal pressures to conform. Yet, building and nurturing strong, healthy relationships is crucial. Surrounding ourselves with people who inspire us, challenge us, and celebrate us as we are can propel us forward on our growth journey.

In fact, a study by Dr. Marisa Franco in *Platonic* shows that our friendships and social connections shape our mental health, boost self-esteem, and even influence our longevity. The connections we forge with others, whether through networking, volunteering, or simply having a safe space with our girls, are pivotal for our personal growth and well-being. Building those relationships where we feel supported and appreciated helps our overall growth.

Spiritual growth plays an essential role in our holistic development. Spirituality isn't confined to religion; it's about connecting with something greater than ourselves and finding meaning and purpose in life. As Black women, we may face spiritual challenges such as feeling disconnected from our culture, spirituality, or community. But we must remember that our roots, our culture, our ancestors, our history, are powerful sources of strength and wisdom.

Spiritual growth involves nourishing our spirit through activities that help us reconnect with our inner self and purpose. This can include practices like meditation, prayer, connecting with our culture, or even fasting for clarity. Fostering inner peace allows us to align with our values and makes us resilient in the face of adversity. Spiritual practices help us to ground ourselves and stay centered as we navigate the world and pursue our goals.

Emotional growth is perhaps one of the most critical aspects of our overall well-being. As Black women, we often face emotional challenges like managing stress, anxiety, and the burden of systemic oppression. However, we are incredibly resilient, and the ability to build emotional intelligence is key to navigating these challenges.

Prioritizing emotional growth means learning how to process our emotions in healthy ways. Practices such as journaling, therapy, mindfulness, and meditation all help in building emotional intelligence. Dr. Sheryl Ziegler's research highlights that emotional resilience plays a critical role in how we cope with stress, bounce back from setbacks, and ultimately succeed in life. It's about gaining awareness of our emotions, learning how to manage them, and cultivating a healthy mindset. By investing time and energy in our emotional health, we strengthen ourselves from the inside out.

Finally, physical growth is essential to our well-being. Nurturing our bodies through exercise, healthy eating, and rest is foundational to supporting every other aspect of growth. By taking care of our physical health, we not only feel better but also have the energy and vitality to tackle the demands of daily life.

Black women, in particular, have a long history of overcoming challenges, and taking care of our physical health ensures we are equipped to continue breaking barriers. Research from the American Heart Association shows that regular physical activity and maintaining a healthy lifestyle reduce the risk of chronic diseases and improve mental health. When we nurture our bodies, we ensure we have the stamina and vitality to face the challenges that life presents while continuing to grow in every other area of our lives.

In order to grow fully, we must prioritize all aspects of ourselves. The key is to embrace the holistic nature of personal growth, integrating mental, social, spiritual, emotional, and physical well-being into our daily lives. Each area supports and nourishes the other, creating a well-rounded approach to self-improvement.

By consciously nurturing these areas, we ensure that we become the best version of ourselves, not only for ourselves but also for the communities we serve, our families, and the generations that follow. Growth is a continuous journey, and as Black women, embracing this journey with positivity and commitment will empower us to rise, not just individually, but as a collective.

Through embracing mental, social, spiritual, emotional, and physical growth, we unlock our fullest potential and create the life we truly deserve. This is the true essence of personal growth: it's not just about becoming better for us but about becoming the women we were always meant to be: powerful, resilient, and ever-evolving.

Setbacks and Growth: The Power of Bouncing Back

Setbacks are inevitable. It's part of the journey. Life will throw curveballs, challenges will emerge, and moments of disappointment will come, but here's the thing: how we respond to them is where the magic happens. It's okay to feel the feels, sis. Take a moment to process the disappointment, the frustration, or the sadness. Feel it. Own it. But, after you've taken that moment, you've got to get back up and keep moving forward. Resilience is all about knowing that every setback, every challenge, is an opportunity to rise higher and stronger than before.

Resilience is absolutely key to personal growth. It's not just about how many times we fall, it's about how many times we get back up. This is where the concept of grit comes into play. Angela Duckworth's pioneering research on grit shows that perseverance, not just intelligence or talent, is the true driver of success. Grit is the combination of passion and perseverance for long-term goals, and it's something that Black women have demonstrated time and time again. In a world that continuously tests our strength, grit is what helps us push through and rise despite the odds.

When we look at historical figures like Madam C.J. Walker, we see the embodiment of grit and resilience. Madam Walker, the first self-made female millionaire in the U.S., built her empire amidst a backdrop of systemic racism, financial hardship, and personal adversity. Her story is a testament to the power of resilience; her determination and vision for success pushed her forward, proving that setbacks are merely stepping stones to achieving greatness. Walker's success didn't come without setbacks, but her ability to persist, adapt, and persevere made her an icon of resilience and empowerment for Black women.

As we navigate our own journeys, let's remember that setbacks don't define us; **they refine us.** Each time we face adversity and rise above it, we become stronger, more determined, and more capable of achieving our dreams. Resilience is a muscle we strengthen every time we overcome a challenge, and by continuing to bounce back, we build a foundation for greater success and fulfillment.

Taking Action

o **Cultivate a Growth Mindset:** Embrace the belief that your abilities and intelligence can be developed through dedication and hard work. Adopting a growth mindset allows you to see challenges as opportunities for learning and growth rather than obstacles to be avoided.

o **Set SMART Goals:** Define specific, measurable, achievable, relevant, and time-bound goals that align with your vision for personal and professional growth. Break down larger goals into smaller, manageable tasks to track your progress and stay motivated.

o **Embrace Discomfort:** Lean into discomfort as a sign of growth and progress. Challenge yourself to step outside of your comfort zone by trying new experiences, taking on unfamiliar tasks, and embracing uncertainty with courage and resilience.

- **Cultivate Resilience:** Develop resilience by viewing setbacks and failures as learning opportunities rather than insurmountable obstacles. Build your resilience muscle by bouncing back from adversity with grace and determination, knowing that setbacks are temporary and can be overcome.

- **Practice Regular Reflection:** Set aside dedicated time for self-reflection to assess your progress, identify areas for improvement, and celebrate your successes. Use journaling, meditation, or conversations with trusted mentors or friends to gain insight into your thoughts, emotions, and behaviors.

- **Seek Feedback and Support:** Surround yourself with a supportive network of friends, mentors, and peers who can offer constructive feedback, encouragement, and guidance on your growth journey. Be open to receiving feedback with humility and gratitude, knowing that it can help you learn and grow.

- **Embrace Lifelong Learning:** Commit to continuous learning and personal development by seeking out opportunities to expand your knowledge, skills, and perspectives. Take courses, attend workshops, read books, and engage in meaningful conversations to deepen your understanding and broaden your horizons.

o **Practice Self-Compassion:** Not too much on yourself, sis! Be gentle and compassionate with yourself as you navigate the ups and downs of growth and self-discovery. Treat yourself with kindness, patience, and understanding, especially during challenging times, and remember that you are worthy of love and acceptance just as you are.

o **Stay Flexible and Adapt:** Remain adaptable and flexible in the face of change, uncertainty, and unexpected obstacles. Embrace the mindset of continuous adaptation and adjustment, knowing that growth often requires flexibility and the willingness to pivot when necessary.

o **Celebrate Your Growth:** Take time to acknowledge and celebrate your growth milestones, even in its most subtle form. Recognize your progress, achievements, and successes along the way, and celebrate the journey of growth and transformation that you are on.

Here are ten affirmations of growth for Black women:

1. I am committed to my personal growth and development.
2. I am open to learning new things and trying new experiences.
3. I embrace challenges as opportunities for growth and learning.
4. I trust in my ability to adapt and overcome obstacles.

5. I am resilient and able to bounce back from setbacks.

6. I am proactive in creating positive changes in my life.

7. I celebrate my progress and achievements, no matter how small they may be.

8. I am patient with myself as I navigate my personal growth journey.

9. I surround myself with people who support and encourage my growth.

10. I am continuously evolving into the best version of myself.

A commitment to continuous learning is the fuel that propels our personal growth. Katherine Johnson, the brilliant NASA mathematician whose calculations helped launch astronauts into space, defied the odds in STEM by relentlessly expanding her knowledge. Her story is a powerful reminder that growth is a never-ending journey, and learning is the key to breaking barriers and seizing new opportunities.

Let's commit wholeheartedly to our growth. Let's invest in ourselves and tap into the limitless power that has always existed within us. Personal growth is not just a destination— it's a lifelong journey that demands patience, dedication, and resilience. It won't always be easy, but the rewards? Oh, they are immeasurable. By prioritizing our growth, we become stronger, more empowered, and more confident in who we are.

As we rise, we also set the stage for others to rise with us. We become living examples of what's possible when we take control of our own narrative. We inspire those around us to embrace their own journeys of self-discovery and empowerment.

So, let's embrace the power of growth. Let's step out of our comfort zones, push past the fear, and become the unapologetic, unstoppable forces we were always destined to be. Together, we can elevate ourselves, our communities, and the world. This is our time to shine as the best versions of ourselves.

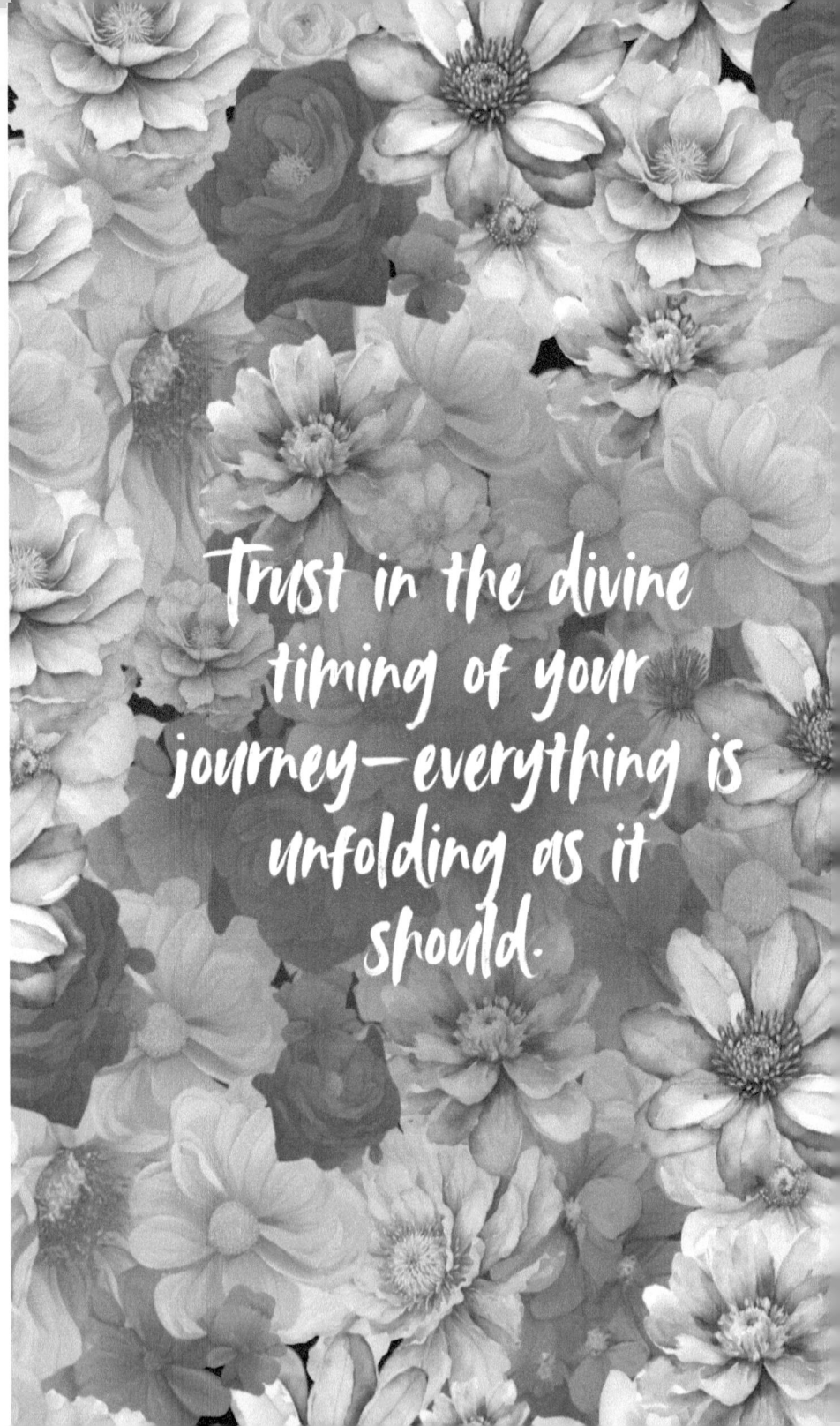

Trust in the divine timing of your journey—everything is unfolding as it should.

7

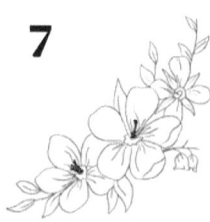

Girl, Just Pray!

Girl,

I do not consider myself super religious, but I believe I know that there is power in prayer. As the saying "God may not come when you want him to, but He is always on time." Prayer is like a lifeline, a direct line to the divine, where you can pour out your heart and soul without fear of judgment

Life can throw some curveballs, can't it? There are moments when it feels like everything is falling apart, and you're left wondering how you'll make it through. But that's where prayer comes in. It's a beacon of hope in the darkness, a reminder that you're never alone, no matter how tough things may seem in the moment

I've experienced firsthand the transformative power of prayer. Most recently, when I was stranded in the airport with my kids, trying to get to New York for a very important contest, prayer brought me comfort in that moment. I had instant clarity that if I didn't make it, it was for a reason, and if, by the grace of God that, I arrived on time, everything was going as planned. I was very stressed, and prayer gave me

Girl, Just Pray!

clarity. Spoiler alert! I made it just in the nick of time! As I was on stage waiting for The UPS Store to announce the winner, I prayed at that moment. Another spoiler, I won!

When life gets tough and you feel like you're at the end of your rope, remember this: just pray. Pour out your heart, and trust that your prayers will be heard. And above all else, have faith that everything will unfold exactly as it should. There is comfort in letting go and letting God.

Stay strong, stay hopeful, and keep prayin'.

Blessings,

The Power of Prayer

In the quiet moments of our lives, there is a profound and transformative power—prayer. Prayer is a timeless practice that transcends cultural boundaries, and for Black women, it serves as a sacred lifeline connecting us to something far greater than ourselves. Prayer is a form of dialogue, a space where we pour our hearts out to the divine, releasing our anxieties, hopes, and gratitude, knowing we are heard.

Dr. Lisa Miller, author of *The Awakened Brain*, discusses how prayer and spiritual connection activate resilience centers in the brain. Her research reveals that this connection enhances emotional regulation and helps us better manage stress, making prayer an invaluable tool for navigating adversity.

For Black women, prayer is not only a source of personal solace but also a method of renewal. When faced with overwhelming obstacles, whether societal, familial, or personal, prayer becomes our refuge, a space where we can ground ourselves and find comfort in the divine. Research by Dr. Thema Bryant-Davis, a psychologist and ordained minister, emphasizes that prayer and faith can work in tandem with therapy to promote holistic healing. It's a dual tool for both the soul and the mind.

Prayer as Self-Care

Self-care goes beyond skincare routines or occasional relaxation; it's about fostering peace in the midst of chaos, and prayer is an essential form of self-care. By expressing gratitude and surrendering our burdens through prayer, we engage in one of the most powerful forms of self-love and healing. Dr. Bryant-Davis underscores that Black women can integrate faith and mental health care to nurture both body and spirit.

Prayer as a Tool for Transformation and Healing

The ability of prayer to transform our hearts and minds cannot be overstated. Whether it's personal challenges, systemic injustices, or the heaviness of everyday life, prayer is an empowering tool that helps Black women stand firm. It gives us the strength to face adversity and the clarity to persevere in the face of hardship.

Take, for example, Fannie Lou Hamer, the civil rights icon who famously used prayer to fuel her fight for justice. Hamer's faith and activism were intricately woven together, as she used prayer to sustain her through some of the most trying moments of her life. Her words, "I'm sick and tired of being sick and tired," remind us that faith is not passive; it's an active force that propels us toward change.

This strength, rooted in prayer, is something Black women have long embodied. From the historical prayers of our ancestors for liberation to the modern-day prayers for justice, Black women's prayers have always been a form of resistance, calling for transformation and healing. Prayer keeps us aligned with our values and fuels our activism, reminding us that our fight for equality and justice is deeply connected to our spiritual strength.

The Divine and Us

Brené Brown's research on vulnerability highlights the significance of showing up fully, imperfectly, and authentically. Prayer is where we do just that. It's where we lay down our insecurities, fears, and doubts, fully trusting that we are loved, accepted, and guided, even when the road is uncertain. Prayer lets us be real, our most vulnerable selves, before the divine without fear of judgment.

Scripture for When Life is Life'n

In those challenging moments when life feels heavy, scripture offers us solace and guidance. The Bible's timeless wisdom speaks directly to the heart of our struggles, offering encouragement, comfort, and direction. The following scriptures are daily reminders to trust the process, find strength in faith, and stay grounded in love:

For Strength and Resilience

"But those who hope in the Lord will renew their strength. They will soar on wings like eagles; they will run and not grow weary; they will walk and not be faint." Isaiah 40:31

For Overcoming Adversity

"And we know that in all things God works for the good of those who love him, who have been called according to his purpose." Romans 8:28

For Finding Peace

"Do not be anxious about anything, but in every situation, by prayer and petition, with thanksgiving, present your requests to God. And the peace of God, which transcends all understanding, will guard your hearts and your minds in Christ Jesus." Philippians 4:6-7

For Guidance and Direction

"Trust in the Lord with all your heart and lean not on your own understanding; in all your ways submit to him, and he will make your paths straight." Proverbs 3:5-6

For Love and Compassion

"Love is patient, love is kind. It does not envy, it does not boast, it is not proud. It does not dishonor others; it is not self-seeking, it is not easily angered, and it keeps no record of wrongs. Love does not delight in evil but rejoices with the truth. It always protects, always trusts, always hopes, always perseveres. Love never fails." 1 Corinthians 13:4-8

For Healing and Restoration

"He heals the brokenhearted and binds up their wounds." Psalm 147:3

For Family and Community

"Let us not become weary in doing good, for at the proper time, we will reap a harvest if we do not give up. Therefore, as we have the opportunity, let us do good to all people, especially to those who belong to the family of believers." Galatians 6:9-10

For Joy and Celebration

"This is the day that the Lord has made; let us rejoice and be glad in it." Psalm 118:24

For Faith and Trust

"Now faith is confidence in what we hope for and assurance about what we do not see." Hebrews 11:1

For Endurance and Perseverance

"Consider it pure joy, my brothers and sisters, whenever you face trials of many kinds, because you know that the testing of your faith produces perseverance. Let perseverance finish its work so that you may be mature and complete, not lacking anything." James 1:2-4

These scriptures remind us that, even in our darkest hours, prayer and faith provide us with the strength, peace, and clarity needed to navigate life's challenges.

Taking Action

Now, let's transform our faith into action! Prayer is more than just a spiritual practice; it's a way to engage with our lives and shape the path ahead actively. Here are a few practical ways to deepen your prayer practice:

o **Establish a Sacred Space:** Designate a peaceful corner or area in your home for prayer and reflection. Surround yourself with things that inspire you—whether it's candles, plants, or meaningful objects. This will be your sanctuary for connection with the divine.

o **Morning Gratitude Routine:** Begin each day with a prayer of gratitude, expressing thanks for the blessings in your life. Take a few moments to reflect on the things you're grateful for, big and small, and offer them up in prayer.

o **Prayer Journaling:** Start a prayer journal to document your thoughts, feelings, and prayers. Use it as a space to pour out your heart to God, write down your hopes and dreams, and reflect on the answers you receive.

o **Prayer Walks:** Incorporate prayer into your daily exercise routine by taking prayer walks in nature. As you walk, express gratitude, ask for guidance, or simply commune with God in the beauty around you.

○ **Prayer Circles:** Form a prayer circle with friends, family, or members of your community. Gather regularly to pray together, share intentions, and support one another spiritually.

○ **Prayer and Meditation Retreat:** Plan a weekend retreat focused on prayer and meditation. Find a peaceful location where you can disconnect from the outside world and immerse yourself in prayer, meditation, and self-reflection.

○ **Service and Prayer:** Combine prayer with acts of service by volunteering in your community or supporting charitable organizations. Use your talents to make a positive impact, and trust that God is guiding your efforts.

○ **Prayer Partnerships:** Pair up with a prayer partner or spiritual mentor to support each other in your prayer lives. Share prayers, offer encouragement, and hold each other accountable for your spiritual growth.

○ **Pray Through Art:** Explore different forms of creative expression, such as painting, drawing, or writing poetry, as a way to connect with God. Use art as a form of prayer, allowing your creativity to flow freely and express your deepest thoughts and emotions.

o **Retreat and Renewal:** Plan a personal retreat focused on prayer and renewal. Take time away from your daily responsibilities to rest, recharge, and reconnect with God. Use this time to recharge your spirit and deepen your prayer practice.

Here are ten affirmations for the praying Black women:

1. I am guided by faith, not fear, trusting in God's divine plan for my life.
2. I am a vessel of God's love, spreading light and compassion wherever I go.
3. I am fearfully and wonderfully made, cherished by the Creator of the universe.
4. I walk in faith, knowing that God's grace is sufficient for me in every circumstance.
5. I am strong and courageous, rooted in the strength of my faith and the power of God's love.
6. I am deserving of God's blessings, and I receive them with gratitude and humility.
7. I am a reflection of God's love and goodness, shining brightly in the world.
8. I am guided by the Holy Spirit, trusting in divine wisdom to lead me on the right path.

9. I am filled with peace and serenity, knowing that God's presence is always with me.

10. I am an instrument of God's peace, bringing hope and healing to those in need.

Let prayer be the foundation upon which you build a life of faith, peace, and transformation. Prayer not only connects us to the divine but also to the collective power of community and sisterhood. As you pray, may you feel the strength of generations before you who used prayer as a tool of resistance and empowerment.

Let's make prayer a part of our daily practice and watch how it transforms not just our lives but the lives of those around us. Stay strong, stay hopeful, and know that the divine is always listening. We are never alone. Keep praying, keep believing, and keep shining.

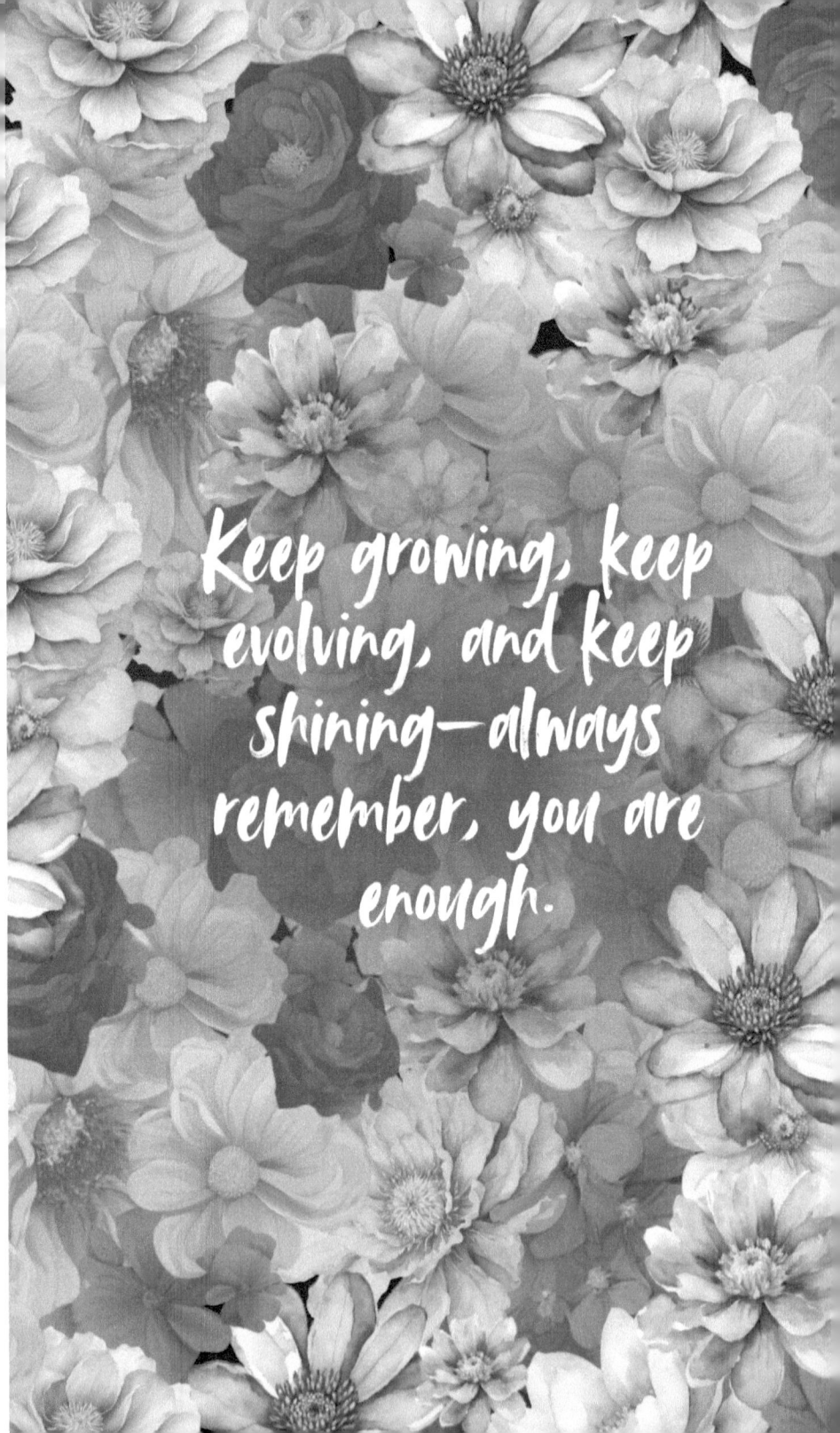

Keep growing, keep evolving, and keep shining—always remember, you are enough.

Final Word:
You are Magical!

Dear Black Woman,

If you don't remember anything else, remember this. You don't owe anyone anything. You are enough! You are amazing! I am in awe of the melanin beauty that is you!

With love and admiration,

P.S. Keep shining bright!

Black girl magic isn't just a term; it's a powerful way of life. It encapsulates the certitude, strength, and beauty that Black women exude every day. It's the incredible ability to turn obstacles into triumphs, challenges into opportunities. At its core, Black girl magic is about self-belief and recognizing the immense power that comes with being a Black woman.

To tap into your Black girl magic, you must first believe in yourself and your abilities. Know that your Blackness is not a limitation but a powerful source of magic and strength. Black women have always been at the forefront of change, fighting for justice equality, and breaking down barriers. It's this same perseverance and determination that makes Black women magical.

Overcoming adversity is at the heart of Black girl magic. From fighting for civil rights to demanding equality in every corner of life, Black women have faced hurdles that would have broken others. Yet, time and time again, Black women have stood tall and persevered. Their tenacity is not just admirable; it's magical.

Shining bright is another defining trait of Black girl magic. Society has long taught Black women to dim their light to make others comfortable. But Black girl magic is about embracing your uniqueness and unapologetically letting your light shine. Whether it's in fashion, art, careers, or entrepreneurship, Black women are breaking boundaries and making waves across every industry.

As Auntie Tab, the one and only Mrs. Tabitha Brown, has so eloquently shared, she spent years shrinking herself to fit into the expectations of others. But as she's learned, and as we all must embrace, other people's comfort is *not* our problem. Never dim your light to make others comfortable.

We've spent too long conforming, probably code-switching, without even thinking about it. That time is over. It's time to shine unapologetically. Dr. Joan Morgan, in her groundbreaking work *When Chickenheads Come Home to Roost*, challenges us to redefine Black womanhood on our own terms. Hip-hop feminism teaches us that we don't have to choose between softness and strength, career and creativity, tradition and innovation—we can embody all of it, and we can do it fearlessly. Here's your permission (that you don't need, by the way): You don't have to sprinkle your magic everywhere, but you do get to embrace your authentic self and shine fully without reservation.

Did you catch the big ideas throughout this book? In all your magic, it's vital to stay grounded in gratitude, have a strong support system, set healthy boundaries, practice self-compassion, prioritize self-care, celebrate your wins, and be resilient.

To help you embrace your magic unapologetically, we've created the *Black Girl Magic Principles*. These principles serve as the essence of empowerment and self-love. Embrace them as your guide to living out your magic unapologetically and authentically.

Black Girl Magic Principles

I.   Cultivate a mindset of gratitude, appreciating the blessings and lessons in your life.

II.   Surround yourself with a supportive network of friends, family, and mentors who uplift and empower you.

III.   Set healthy boundaries to protect your energy, time, and well-being from negative influences.

IV.   Practice self-compassion by treating yourself with kindness, understanding, and forgiveness.

V.   Prioritize self-care activities that nourish your mind, body, and soul, ensuring you are refreshed and rejuvenated.

VI.   Celebrate your accomplishments, milestones, and unique qualities, embracing your worth and value.

VII.   Cultivate resilience by facing challenges with courage, perseverance, and a positive mindset.

VIII.   Above all, give yourself grace, recognizing that you are human and deserving of love, compassion, and acceptance.

Having a sense of purpose is the foundation of Black girl magic. Knowing that you have a purpose, and using your unique gifts to fulfill it is the ultimate expression of magic. It's about recognizing that your talents are not just for personal success but for making a meaningful difference in the world. When you embrace your purpose, you leave a lasting legacy that empowers others and uplifts communities.

Affirmations for Black Girl Magic:

1. My Blackness is a source of magic and power.
2. I am worthy of success and happiness.
3. I embrace my uniqueness and use it to shine bright.
4. I am capable of achieving anything I set my mind to.
5. I am resilient in the face of adversity and challenges.
6. My beauty is not limited by societal standards.
7. I am a force to be reckoned with.
8. My presence and voice matter.
9. I honor my ancestors and their sacrifices.
10. I am grateful for the gift of being a Black woman.

Black girl magic is about celebrating the beauty, strength, and self-reliance of Black women. And that's on PERIOD. It's about recognizing our worth, honoring our power, and using it to create meaningful change in the world. Black girl magic isn't just a phrase; it's a way of life. It's about embracing the unique qualities that make you and using them to make an impact that ripples through time.

Black women are magical, and our magic will continue to inspire future generations of Black girls to come.

You are magic, sis! Black girl magic is real, and you carry it with you every single day. As Maya Angelou beautifully declared in *Phenomenal Woman*, there is power in your walk, your presence, and the way you command space. This magic isn't about being perfect; it's about the undeniable brilliance and strength that radiates from being a Black woman, a legacy that has been passed down from our ancestors and carried forward through every triumph we claim today.

This book is just the beginning. Keep growing, keep shining. As Toni Morrison once said, "You are your best thing." Let that be your guiding principle: honor your worth, celebrate your joy, and never forget that you are magic in every form, in every moment.

Acknowledgements

So Much Thanks to Give

I have so much to be thankful for and so many that I appreciate for being a part of the reason that this became a reality. I'd like to thank my support system for making this possible. Without my mom, friends, and other family, this would not have been possible. Two ladies, Serritha Johnson and Rosetta M.C., who are also fellow authors, motivated me to finish this project I started long ago. I had the pleasure of reading both of their books, which are also listed in the resources section.

My husband and my girls, Skylar and Danielle, have been so patient with me as I have dedicated more and more time to building and nurturing Ebony Notes to be as great as it can be.

Thank you to two women whose relationships started in a space all about business, but y'all have become two of my closest friends, Kalea and Anita. Y'all have become so much more than cheerleaders for Ebony Notes; y'all support LaDonna, the person, when I just needed a listening ear or a shoulder for support.

Kalea once said, "I think you can just say your friend now," while I was searching for the words to describing who I was having a meal with to my brother. We lowkey became a little co-dependent, in a good way, the way we text and talk almost daily.

Anita, Anita, Anita. I appreciate your perspective always and how you stand on your convictions. Who else is doing 3 hours, both ways turn and burn, to support my event? When it comes to these money numbers, business or personal, she's standing on business.

On the subject of all business, thank you to a sister I didn't know I needed, Amber Joy Simon. You have been so encouraging and helpful throughout my Ebony Notes journey and teaching me about living a pleasure first life. The way you hype me up, it's undeniable. I can just hear you saying, "Come on now, sis." in your voice in my head, and it makes me smile and keep on pushing to do whatever thing I'm struggling with at the time.

I have an immense amount of respect and gratitude for my aunt, Dr. Danyell Crutchfield-Cummings. Not only did she, as busy as she is, contribute to this book, but I've always looked up to her in such a special way. She is one of the reasons I landed in education and always aspired to do and be more. If no one else showed up, she did, and that meant something to me. We do not talk on a regular basis, but if I call, text, or email with a need, she is there to support me in whatever the endeavor may be. She is the only family member besides my mother who rocks with me like that. For always making me feel seen and heard when I felt that no one saw or heard, thank you Auntie!

There are so many of y'all riding for me and rooting for me to win each and every time. If you aren't mentioned by name, charge it to my mind, not my heart.

Another group that played a huge role in the fulfillment of this book is the Early Reader Sisters. Thank you to all of my Early Reader Sisters. This is the group who took the time to read my book and give invaluable feedback along the way. I want to thank each and every one of them for taking the time to read the book and give meaningful feedback.

Thank you to:

Serritha Johnson

And several others who left anonymous feedback.

Here's a little of what Serritha had to say:

"This book is soul medicine. Ebony Notes for Black Women is exactly what we need in a world that often pits Black women against each other—on social media, through relationships, cultural messaging, and more. From the first page, LaDonna reminds us of the beauty and brilliance of being a Black queen. She doesn't just tell us to heal—she shows us how. Through daily affirmations, loving self-talk, and real action steps, she gives us tools to unlearn harmful messages and walk in wholeness. One of my favorite quotes? "Listen up, beautiful: forgiving doesn't mean forgetting... it's about releasing yourself from the burden of carrying around all that pain." It feels like a deep conversation with your most trusted friend. LaDonna is the real deal. She helped me publish my own book, leads the wellness program at our school, and is actively building a real-life community for Black women in our city. She lives what she writes.

Do yourself a favor and GET THIS BOOK! You'll grow, heal, and feel seen." - Serritha Johnson

Glossary

Affirmations – Positive statements that help reprogram the subconscious mind to reinforce confidence and self-worth.

Affirmative Prayer – A spiritual practice that focuses on expressing gratitude and positivity, and affirming one's desires as already being fulfilled.

Body Scan- a mindfulness meditation technique that involves paying attention to your body and noticing sensations without judgment.

Cultural Resilience – The ability of a group, particularly marginalized communities, to resist and bounce back from societal, racial, or cultural adversity while preserving their traditions and identity.

Divine Feminine – A spiritual concept representing nurturing, intuition, and creative energy, often associated with goddesses like Oshun.

Empowerment – The process of gaining confidence, control, and strength, often in relation to overcoming adversity or societal expectations. It involves asserting one's rights and pursuing one's goals with courage.

Energy Healing – A holistic practice focused on balancing and restoring the body's energy systems to promote physical and emotional well-being, often through practices like Reiki or crystal healing.

Goddess Energy – A term used to describe the power, resilience, and grace Black women embody.

Growth Mindset – A psychological belief that abilities, intelligence, and self-perception can evolve through effort and learning (coined by Dr. Carol Dweck).

Healing – The process of overcoming emotional, physical, or psychological trauma and restoring balance, health, and well-being.

Holistic Healing – An approach to wellness that considers the whole person—mind, body, and spirit—rather than just treating symptoms or physical illness.

Inner Goddess – The essence of self-love, self-worth, and personal power that all women possess.

Mindfulness – The practice of being fully present in the moment and observing thoughts, feelings, and sensations without judgment. It is often used as a technique for managing stress and enhancing emotional well-being.

Oshun – One of the most well-known Yoruba Orishas, represents divine femininity, love, beauty, and abundance. In Yoruba culture, she is honored as a source of grace, sensuality, and healing.

Resilience – The ability to overcome adversity and continue to grow despite challenges.

Radical Self-Acceptance – The practice of embracing all parts of oneself, including imperfections, without judgment and living authentically and unapologetically.

Sacred Feminine – A term that honors the divine feminine qualities such as compassion, creativity, intuition, and nurturing within all women and the world.

Sacred Space – A physical or mental space that holds deep spiritual meaning, where an individual can retreat to for peace, reflection, or prayer.

Self-Care – The practice of taking time to care for your mental, emotional, and physical health. It includes activities that replenish your energy and maintain your well-being.

Self-Compassion – The practice of treating oneself with kindness, care, and understanding in the face of difficulties or mistakes, as coined by Dr. Kristin Neff.

Self-Perception – How an individual views themselves, including their confidence, self-worth, and abilities.

Sisterhood – A supportive, empowering bond between women, especially among Black women, that emphasizes mutual care, upliftment, and shared experiences.

Spiritual Awakening – The process of becoming more aware of one's spiritual nature, purpose, and connection to the universe or divine.

Spiritual Wellness – The integration of spiritual practices and values that nurture personal growth, healing, and alignment with one's higher purpose.

Yoruba – The Yoruba people are one of the largest ethnic groups in West Africa, primarily found in Nigeria, Benin, and Togo. Yoruba spirituality is rich with mythology, deities (Orisha), and traditions that emphasize balance, destiny, and personal power.

References

Books & Articles:

Angelou, M. (2008). *Letter to My Daughter.* Random House.

Bradford, J. H. (2021). *Sisterhood Heals: The Transformative Power of Black Women's Friendships.* Hay House.

Bryant-Davis, T. (2019). *Thriving in the Wake of Trauma: A Multicultural Guide to Healing and Empowerment.* Routledge.

Bryant-Davis, T. (2022). *Homecoming: Overcome Fear and Trauma to Reclaim Your Whole, Authentic Self.* TarcherPerigee.

Brown, B. (2012). *Daring Greatly: How the Courage to Be Vulnerable Transforms the Way We Live, Love, Parent, and Lead.* Penguin Random House.

Cohn, M. A., Fredrickson, B. L., Brown, S. L., Mikels, J. A., & Conway, A. M. (2014). Happiness unpacked: Positive emotions increase life satisfaction by building resilience. *Psychology of Well-Being, 4*(1), 9.

References

DeGruy, J. (2005). *Post-Traumatic Slave Syndrome: America's Legacy of Enduring Injury and Healing.* Uptone Press.

Duckworth, A. (2016). *Grit: The Power of Passion and Perseverance.* Scribner.

Dweck, C. (2006). *Mindset: The New Psychology of Success.* Random House.

Franco, M. G. (2022). *Platonic: How the Science of Attachment Can Help You Make—and Keep—Friends.* Hachette Books.

Goleman, D. (1995). *Emotional Intelligence: Why It Can Matter More Than IQ.* Bantam.

Hamer, F. L. (1967). "I'm sick and tired of being sick and tired," Testimony at the Democratic National Convention.

hooks, bell. (2000). *All About Love: New Visions.* William Morrow Paperbacks.

Hurston, Z. N. (2006). *Dust Tracks on a Road.* Harper Perennial Modern Classics.

Lorde, A. (1984). *Sister Outsider: Essays and Speeches.* Crossing Press.

McClain, T. (2019). *The Legacy of Madam C.J. Walker: Resilience and Success Against the Odds.* African American Entrepreneurship Journal, 11(2), 120-135.

Miller, L. (2021). *The Awakened Brain: The New Science of Spirituality and Our Quest for an Inspired Life.* St. Martin's Press.

Morgan, J. (2006). *When Chickenheads Come Home to Roost: A Hip-Hop Feminist Breaks It Down.* Touchstone.

Rae, I. (2016). "I'm rooting for everybody Black." [Red carpet interview]. In *2017 Golden Globe Awards.*

Tatum, B. D. (2017). *Why Are All the Black Kids Sitting Together in the Cafeteria?* Basic Books.

Walker, C. J. (2001). *On Her Own Ground: The Life and Times of Madam C.J. Walker.* Scribner.

Wilkins, A. (2020). The Role of African Spirituality in the Emotional and Psychological Healing of African American Women. *International Journal of African American Studies, 23*(1), 1-15.

Ziegler, S. (2019). The Importance of Emotional Resilience in Overcoming Adversity. *Journal of Emotional Well-Being.*

References

Music:

Beyoncé. (2022). *Cozy.* On *Renaissance.* Parkwood Entertainment/Columbia Records.

India.Arie. (2001). *Video.* On *Acoustic Soul.* Motown Records.

Kendrick Lamar. (2017). *DNA.* On *DAMN.* Top Dawg Entertainment.

Websites:

Therapy for Black Girls. (n.d.). *Find a therapist.* Retrieved from https://therapyforblackgirls.com

Henson, T. P. (2018). *The Boris Lawrence Henson Foundation.* Retrieved from https://borislhensonfoundation.org

Scientific Journals:

Cohn, M. A., Fredrickson, B. L., Brown, S. L., Mikels, J. A., & Conway, A. M. (2014). Happiness unpacked: Positive emotions increase life satisfaction by building resilience. *Emotion, 12*(5), 92-95. https://doi.org/10.1037/a0038171

Berridge, K. C., & Robinson, T. E. (2003). Parsing reward. *Trends in Neurosciences, 26*(9), 507–513. https://doi.org/10.1016/S0166-2236(03)00233-8

Resources

There are several tools in the **Ebony Notes Co** ecosystem, which include identity-based affirmations, guided journaling, audio series, and meditations.

- **The Ebony Notes App** – Includes identity-based affirmations, guided journaling, audio series, and meditations designed to support mental wellness, self-love, and personal growth. The app is a comprehensive tool that empowers users to take charge of their wellness journey through practical and spiritually aligned features.

- **Journals/Planners** – Custom-designed journals and planners that guide users through reflective writing exercises, goal-setting, and gratitude practices. These journals are crafted to support mental clarity, emotional release, and self-discovery, helping users align their thoughts with their values and intentions.

- **Digital Tools** – A range of digital resources, including templates, printable worksheets, planners, and affirmation cards, are designed to help individuals track their progress, set intentions, and stay focused on their growth journey. These tools can be used alongside the app or as stand-alone resources for a deeper self-care practice.

- **Wellness Community** – An online space where users can connect, share experiences, support one another, and participate in group challenges. This community fosters a sense of belonging, empowerment, and collective growth, where like-minded individuals come together to celebrate and encourage each other's journeys toward wellness.

Therapist Directories

- Therapy for Black Girls – A directory for finding culturally competent therapists. https://therapyforblackgirls.com/
- Black Female Therapists (BFT) – A directory and community highlighting Black women therapists and wellness professionals. https://www.blackfemaletherapists.com/
- Inclusive Therapists – A directory focused on connecting people of color, LGBTQ+ individuals, and other marginalized communities with affirming mental health providers. https://www.inclusivetherapists.com/
- Open Path Collective – A national directory offering affordable mental health care with therapists providing reduced-rate sessions. https://openpathcollective.org/

- Melanin & Mental Health – A resource that connects Black and Latinx individuals to culturally competent therapists and wellness professionals. https://www.melaninandmentalhealth.com/
- Clinicians of Color – A nationwide directory that highlights Black, Indigenous, and people of color (BIPOC) mental health professionals. https://www.cliniciansofcolor.org/
- Zencare – A therapist directory that allows users to watch introductory videos of therapists, making it easier to find the right fit. https://www.zencare.co/
- National Queer and Trans Therapists of Color Network (NQTTCN) – A healing justice organization that connects queer and trans people of color with mental health practitioners. https://www.nqttcn.com/

Mental Health Financial Assistance

- The Loveland Foundation Therapy Fund – Provides financial assistance and access to therapy services for Black women and girls. https://thelovelandfoundation.org/
- Black Girls Smile Therapy Assistance Program – Offers therapy scholarships covering 2 to 6 months of therapy sessions for Black girls and young women. https://www.blackgirlssmile.org/therapy-scholarship

- BEAM (Black Emotional and Mental Health Collective) Grants – Provides grants and financial aid to individuals, collectives, and organizations to support mental health and wellness. https://beam.community/grants/

- BIPOC Therapy Fund – Offers financial support for mental health therapy to Black, Indigenous, and People of Color (BIPOC) adults in the U.S. who are seeking therapy for the first time. https://mentalhealthliberation.org/bipoc-therapy-fund/

- Medicaid Mental Health Services – A federal and state program that provides health coverage, including mental health services, for eligible low-income individuals. https://www.medicaid.gov/medicaid/benefits/behavioral-health-services/index.html

- Sliding Scale Therapy Clinics – Many mental health clinics offer sliding scale fees based on income. Use the HRSA Health Center Locator to find local community health clinics that provide low-cost therapy services. https://findahealthcenter.hrsa.gov/

- SAMHSA Treatment Services Locator – A nationwide database of mental health and substance use treatment facilities that offer payment assistance or sliding scale fees. https://findtreatment.samhsa.gov/

- NAMI (National Alliance on Mental Illness) Financial Assistance for Mental Health – Information on financial support options for mental health care, including SSI (Supplemental Security Income) and SSDI (Social Security Disability Insurance). https://www.nami.org/Your-Journey/Individuals-with-Mental-Illness/Understanding-Health-Insurance/Paying-for-Care

- FindHelp.org – Local Financial Assistance – A searchable database for finding local financial assistance programs, including mental health support, rent relief, and utility aid. https://www.findhelp.org/

- Open Path Collective – A nonprofit organization that provides access to affordable, sliding-scale therapy for individuals who cannot afford standard rates. https://openpathcollective.org/

Apps & Tools

- Shine App – A meditation and self-care app designed for Black women and women of color.

- The Pattern – A personal growth and astrology-based app that provides insights on self-awareness.

- My Affirmations: Live Positive – Helps you create and schedule affirmations to reinforce positive thinking.

Support Groups & Communities

- Black Women's Health Imperative – Focuses on health and wellness support for Black women. https://bwhi.org/
- The Nap Ministry – Encourages rest as a form of resistance and self-care for Black women. https://thenapministry.com/
- The Black Girl Social Club – A global community fostering sisterhood, networking, and empowerment for Black women.
- https://theblackgirlsocialclub.com/
- Black Girls Brunch - Focused on helping women discover new places, connect with like-minded individuals, and thrive through social events, primarily centered around brunch. https://www.brownskinbrunchin.com/
- Exhale - Inclusive mental and emotional well-being app that centers Black Women, providing support for the unique stressors we face. https://www.exhale-app.com/

Book Recommendations

- After the Rain: Gentle Reminders for Healing, Courage, and Self-Love by Alexandra Elle (2020)

A beautifully written collection of affirmations and reminders for Black women to embrace self-love, healing, and courage.

- A Renaissance of Our Own: A Memoir & Manifesto on Reimagining by Rachel Cargle (2023)

  A thought-provoking memoir and manifesto offering new perspectives on self-empowerment, identity, and reimagining the future.

- Feeding the Soul (Because It's My Business): Finding Our Way to Joy, Love, and Freedom by Tabitha Brown

  A heartfelt guide from Tabitha Brown on finding joy, love, and freedom through self-discovery and self-care.

- Girl, Get Off the Couch by Dr. Radisha Brown

  A motivational book designed to inspire and empower women to break free from fear, overcome obstacles, and take action in their lives.

- Love Languages of God by Serritha Johnson

An insightful exploration of how different people experience and give love, emphasizing the divine connection to our individual love languages.

- Morgan, Joan. When Chickenheads Come Home to Roost: A Hip-Hop Feminist Breaks It Down (1999)

  A groundbreaking work of hip-hop feminism where Joan Morgan breaks down Black womanhood, identity, and empowerment in a new light.

- Self-Care Affirmations for Black Women by Rosetta M.C.

  A collection of affirmations specifically crafted to empower and uplift Black women, promoting healing and self-care practices.

- Walk Through Fire: A Memoir of Love, Loss, and Triumph by Sheila Johnson

  A powerful memoir chronicling Sheila Johnson's journey of overcoming loss, embracing strength, and finding healing through love and resilience.

- When Chickenheads Come Home to Roost: A Hip-Hop Feminist Breaks It Down by Joan Morgan (1999)

Morgan's critical work on Black womanhood, hip-hop culture, and the intersections of race, gender, and identity.

- You Are a Badass by Jen Sincero

  A motivational book about taking charge of your life, achieving your goals, and embracing your personal power to create the life you desire.

- The Four Agreements: A Practical Guide to Personal Freedom by Don Miguel Ruiz

  A spiritual classic offering four guiding principles to create personal freedom and peace.

- The Gifts of Imperfection by Brené Brown

  A guide to embracing vulnerability, letting go of perfectionism, and cultivating self-compassion for personal growth and joy.

- The Power of Now: A Guide to Spiritual Enlightenment by Eckhart Tolle

  A transformative book teaching the importance of living in the present moment and freeing ourselves from the constraints of the mind.

- Black Feminist Thought by Patricia Hill Collins

  A foundational text in understanding the intersections of race, gender, and class within Black feminist theory and its importance in social justice movements.

- I Am That Girl: How to Speak Your Truth, Discover Your Purpose, and Live a Life You Love by Alexis Jones

  A motivational book that encourages women to speak their truth and live authentically in a world full of distractions.

- The Body Is Not an Apology: The Power of Radical Self-Love by Sonya Renee Taylor

  A guide to embracing body positivity and practicing radical self-love for personal and collective healing.

- Women Who Run With the Wolves by Clarissa Pinkola Estés

  A deep dive into the stories of wild women, reclaiming feminine power and wisdom through myths, tales, and psychological insights.

- Radical Self-Love: A Guide to Loving Yourself and Living Your Truth by Gala Darling

  A bold and empowering book encouraging readers to practice self-love and authenticity as tools for transforming their lives.

Meditation Tools

- Zee Clark: https://www.youtube.com/c/ZeeClarke
- Kickin It With Ki - Cut The Noise: https://www.youtube.com/@kickinitwithki-cutthenoise9365

Podcasts for Mental Wellness & Growth

- Therapy for Black Girls – Dr. Joy Harden Bradford.
- The Homecoming Podcast with Dr. Thema Bryant – Addresses healing from trauma and reclaiming self-worth.
- Balanced Black Girl Podcast – Hosted by Lestraundra Alfred – Focuses on wellness and self-improvement for Black women.
- The Friend Zone Podcast – Covers mental health, wellness, and pop culture through a Black lens.
- For Harriet (YouTube Channel) – Engages in conversations around Black women's identity, empowerment, and history.

- Black Girl Burnout - Healing, joy, and abundance

Social Media Influencers & Thought Leaders

- Tabitha Brown (@iamtabithabrown) – Joy, mindfulness, and balance.
- Alexandra Elle (@alex_elle) – Self-care, healing, and journaling.
- The Nap Ministry (@thenapministry) – Rest and resistance.
- Saved in the City (@savedinthecity) - Women, faith, and community

About the Author

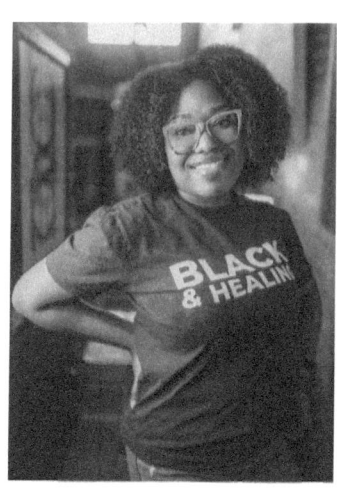

LaDonna Welch is a visionary leader dedicated to promoting mental wellness and self-care within the Black community. She is a multi-talented individual with a diverse background in education, technology, and wellness. As an educator and military spouse, she has a strong sense of community and the importance of supporting those in need. Her experience teaching coding and robotics to students of all ages has given her a unique perspective on how technology can be used to promote education and personal growth. LaDonna's passion for mental health and wellness led her to create Ebony Notes Company, a company dedicated to promoting self-care and well-being within the Black community. LaDonna's expertise in technology and programming languages and diverse interests have been integral to developing the Ebony Notes mobile app. As the founder of Ebony Notes, LaDonna is committed to positively impacting the Black community and beyond with affirmations, stationery, and resources for personal growth. Her dedication to providing multigenerational wellness and mental health support has created a unique and valuable resource for the Black community.

As a visionary leader in the field of mental wellness advocacy, LaDonna Welch's innovative strategies and commitment to empowerment have earned her recognition in multiple local media outlets across Louisiana, Colorado, and Arkansas. LaDonna has also been featured in prestigious publications such as AfroTech and Inc. Magazine. In addition, she was awarded the 2023 Small Biz Challenge by The UPS Store. Through Ebony Notes, LaDonna continues to make a significant impact by providing culturally sensitive resources and support for personal growth and well-being.